Self–assessment Picture Tests

Gastroenterology

second edition

Self-assessment Picture Tests

Gastroenterology

second edition

Miles C. Allison
MD MRCP

Consultant Gastroenterologist
Department of Adult Medicine
Royal Gwent Hospital
Newport
South Wales

M Mosby-Wolfe

London • Baltimore • Barcelona • Bogotá • Boston
Buenos Aires • Carlsbad, CA • Chicago • Madrid
Mexico City • Milan • Naples, FL • New York
Philadelphia • St. Louis • Seoul • Singapore
Sydney • Taipei • Tokyo • Toronto • Wiesbaden

Publisher:	**Richard Furn**
Project Manager:	**Katie Pattullo**
Index:	**Angela Cottingham**
Design:	**Greg Smith**

Published in 1997 by Mosby, an imprint of Times Mirror International Publishers Limited

Printed by Vincenzo Bona s.r.l., Turin, Italy.

ISBN : 0-7234-2589-2

For full details of all Times Mirror International Publishers Limited titles, please write to Times Mirror International Publishers Limited, Lynton House, 7–12 Tavistock Square, London WC1H 9LB, England.

A CIP catalogue record for this book is available from the British Library.

Preface

Diseases of the gastrointestinal tract and liver are encountered commonly by practitioners in most branches of medicine. The wide variety of associated symptoms and signs may lead to initial consultations with family practitioners, physicians, general surgeons, infectious disease specialists, dermatologists, ophthalmologists and many others. The gastroenterologist cannot practice effectively without support from colleagues in fields such as surgery, radiology and the many branches of pathology. It is hoped that trainees and specialists in these diverse disciplines will agree that the Self-assessment Picture Test format is an informative and enjoyable way to tour the various diseases of the gut and liver.

Some of the illustrations demand simple spot diagnoses and questions on associated diseases. Others require more complex interpretation of clinical information and results of diagnostic investigations. Nearly all of the common disorders of the gut and liver are covered, and many rarer conditions are also included. The repertoire of picture tests is thus designed to suit those studying for either undergraduate or postgraduate examinations. This book is intended to illustrate and supplement the fundamental knowledge acquired from standard lectures and textbooks. Moreover, it may come as a refreshing change to those heavily embroiled in preparing for examinations by these conventional means!

The important contributions of diagnostic and therapeutic endoscopy have revolutionised the practice of gastroenterology in recent years. Many potential applications of endoscopy have been covered in this text. Recent refinements in endoscopic imaging have enabled gastroenterology to become an ever more colourful specialty!

Miles C. Allison

Acknowledgements

I would like to thank the many people who have helped me collect so many slides during the last 10 years. In particular I wish to thank Professor Roy Pounder and Dr Paul Dhillon. Roy launched me on the pathway of colour atlases and Paul has spent a lot of time photographing gross and microscopic pathological specimens for our collaborative efforts. I am also grateful for the help given by those in the Medical Illustration departments at the Royal Free Hospital, The Royal Gwent Hospital and Glasgow Royal Infirmary.

Those who have contributed images for this book are: Dr S Lucas (**19**), Mrs A Smith (**39**), Mr H B Torrance (**63**, **115**), Dr C Farthing (**67**), Dr R Clements (**69**, **140**), Professor Dame Sheila Sherlock (**95**, **188**, **191**), Dr A J W Hilson (**106**), Dr D Nicholson (**121**), Dr E Sweet (**127**), Dr M Bernard (**131**, **193**), Mr F Speirs (**139**, **159**), Dr R I Russell (**152**), Professor P-J Lamey (**161**), Dr P Chiodini (**166**, **167**), Professor C D Forbes (**181**, **192**), Dr S K Goolamali (**187**).

QUESTIONS

QUESTIONS

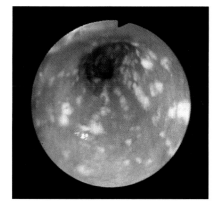

◄ **1, 2** This was the endoscopic appearance of the oesophagus in a 25-year-old man with pain on swallowing. The appearances on oesophageal biopsy are shown in **2**.
(a) What is the diagnosis?
(b) Give three possible predisposing factors.

◄ **2**

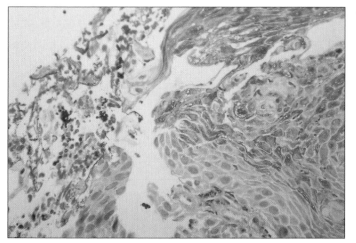

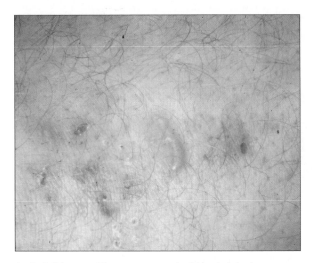

▲ **3** A 34-year-old man presented with a rash and severe itching of the elbows and forearms.
(a) What is the lesion?
(b) How could this diagnosis be confirmed?
(c) Which gastroenterological disorder may be associated?

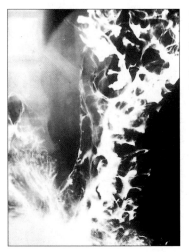

◄ **4** This barium meal radiograph was from a 52-year-old woman with long-standing dyspepsia who had recently developed peripheral oedema.
(a) Which rare condition is present?
(b) Why did she develop oedema?

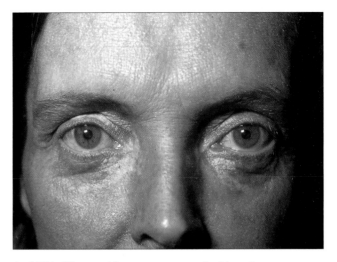

▲ **5** This 57-year-old woman presented with ascites.
(a) Give three abnormalities.
(b) What is the diagnosis?
(c) What form of treatment should be considered in order to improve her survival prospects?

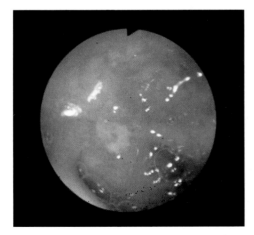

◄ **6** This ulcer was found in the third part of the duodenum on endoscopic examination of a 60-year-old man with melaena stool. Give two possible causes for an ulcer at this unusual site.

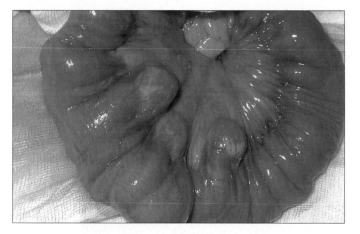

▲ 7 The small intestine of an elderly woman is displayed at laparotomy.
(a) What abnormality is shown?
(b) Give two possible complications.

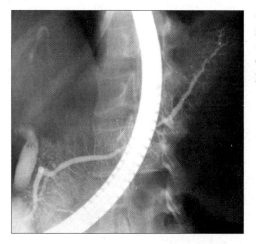

◀ 8 (a) What investigation is being performed?
(b) Give two possible complications of this procedure.

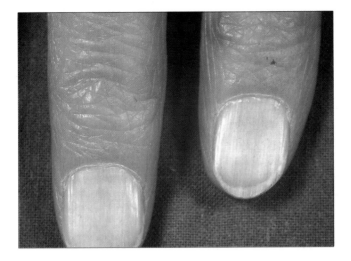

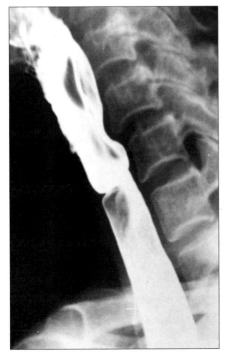

▲ 9, 10 These fingers are from a woman who presented with brittle nails. The pharyngeal region is shown by the barium meal radiograph in 10.
(a) Why were her nails brittle?
(b) What abnormality is seen on the radiograph?
(c) What complication may develop in the pharyngeal region?

◄ 10

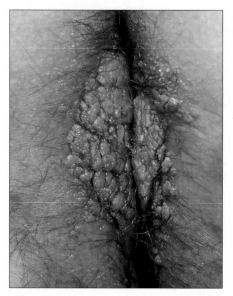

◀ **11** (a) What abnormality is present at the anal region?
(b) Which aetiological agent has been implicated?

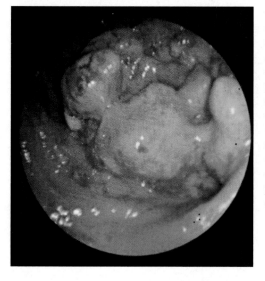

◀ **12** This colonoscopic appearance was found in a 35-year-old man with a 2-month history of colicky central abdominal pain. No other abnormality was noted at colonoscopy.
(a) What abnormality is shown?
(b) Which inherited disorder may have predisposed to this condition?

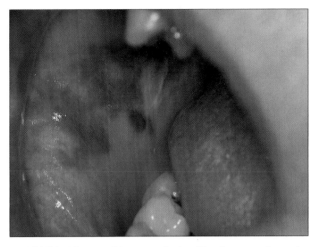

▲ **13** This 30-year-old woman had suffered repeated attacks of diarrhoea, vomiting and abdominal pain. She had lost 7 kg in weight over 1 year.
(a) What is the diagnosis?
(b) How is this confirmed?

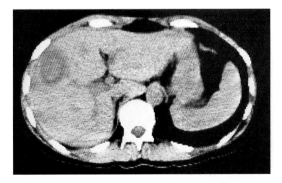

▲ **14** This computerized tomographic (CT) scan was from a 42-year-old woman with fever and right upper quadrant pain. She had returned from Kenya 3 months previously.
(a) What abnormality is noted in the liver?
(b) What is the most likely diagnosis?
(c) How is this confirmed?
(d) What is the treatment?

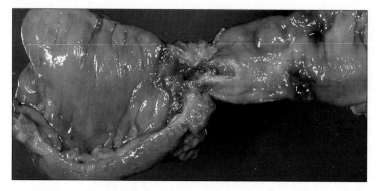

▲ **15** This specimen was resected from the sigmoid colon of a patient with recurrent lower abdominal pain. She had undergone treatment for uterine carcinoma 5 years previously. What is the diagnosis?

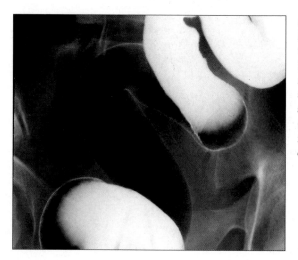

▲ **16** (a) What investigation is this?
(b) What radiological abnormalities are shown?
(c) What is the most likely diagnosis?

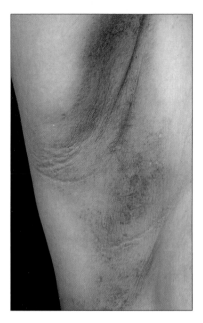

◀ **17** (a) What skin disorder is shown?
(b) Which gastroenterological disorder may be associated?

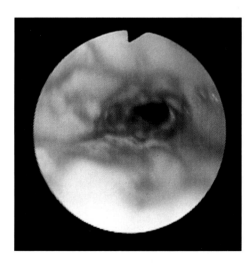

◀ **18** A 78-year-old woman presented with a 2-year history of heartburn, and recent swallowing difficulty.
(a) What abnormalities are seen?
(b) What initial treatment would you recommend?

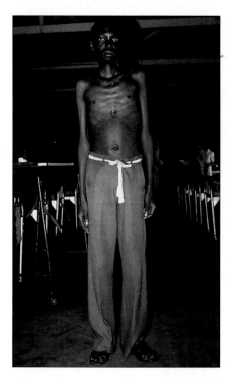

◀ **19, 20** This man presented with weight loss and chronic diarrhoea. The appearances on small bowel biopsy are shown in **20**.
(a) What is the diagnosis?
(b) What is the cause of the diarrhoea?

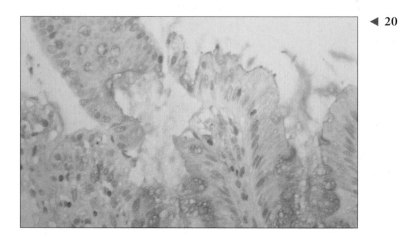

◀ **20**

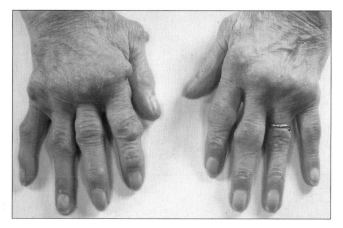

▲ **21, 22** These are the hands of a 70-year-old woman who presented with diarrhoea over several months. A rectal biopsy specimen is shown below in **22.**
(a) What is the main diagnosis?
(b) Why does she have diarrhoea?

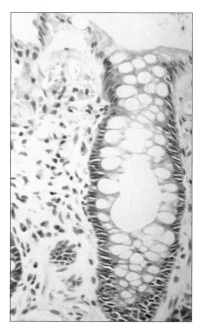

◀ **22**

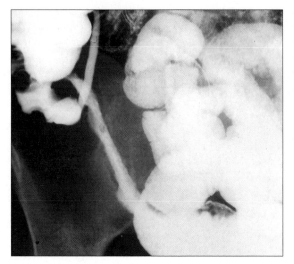

◀ **23** This is a barium follow-through X-ray from a 25-year-old woman with a history of three attacks of severe central abdominal pain and vomiting.
(a) What is the most likely diagnosis?
(b) Give two other diseases which could produce this appearance.

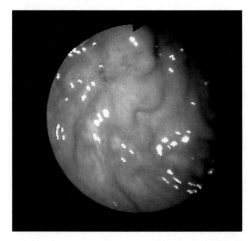

◀ **24** This is an endoscopic photograph of the stomach taken at a level just below the gastro-oesophageal junction from a man who recently had a haematemesis. What abnormality is shown?

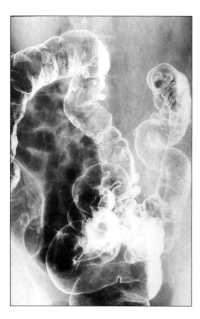

◄ **25** A 69-year-old woman presented with a 2-month history of increased stool frequency, abdominal distension and occasional incontinence of faeces.
(a) What abnormality is shown on this barium enema radiograph?
(b) What is the most likely cause of her symptoms?

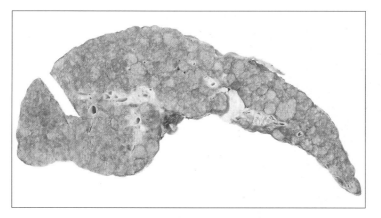

▲ **26** This is the postmortem appearance of liver from an elderly woman who had died after an acute upper gastrointestinal haemorrhage.
(a) What feature is demonstrated?
(b) Give three possible aetiological factors for her liver disease.

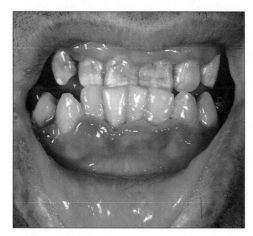

◀ **27** A 27-year-old lorry driver was referred for dietary assessment. Since leaving home he had mainly existed on a diet of peanut butter sandwiches.
(a) What is the cause of the gingival appearances?
(b) Where else would you look for evidence of this disorder?
(c) How is this diagnosis confirmed biochemically?

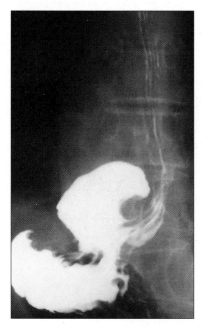

◀ **28** This barium meal radiograph was from a 50-year-old woman with intermittent severe vomiting and swallowing difficulty.
(a) What abnormality is shown?
(b) What treatment should be recommended?

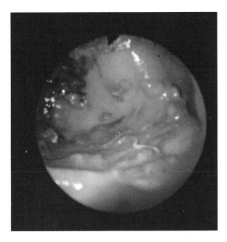

◄ **29** This view was obtained at flexible sigmoidoscopy in a man with severe pruritus ani. What abnormality is present within the rectal lumen?

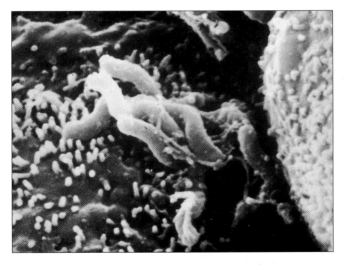

▲ **30** This is a scanning electron micrograph of gastric antral mucosa from a healthy volunteer.
(a) What is this bacterium?
(b) Give four gastric diseases in which it is thought to play an aetiological role.

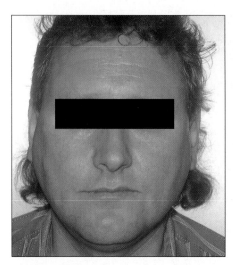

◀ **31** This man was referred for investigation of abnormal biochemical liver function tests.
(a) What abnormality is shown?
(b) What is the probable cause of the liver dysfunction?

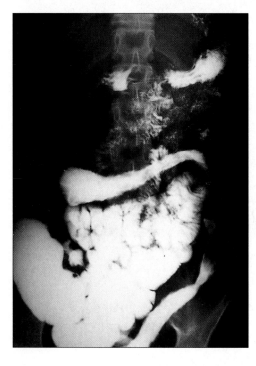

◀ **32** A 25-year-old woman is being investigated for diarrhoea and weight loss. This radiograph was obtained 45 min after ingestion of barium.
(a) What abnormality is demonstrated?
(b) What is the diagnosis?

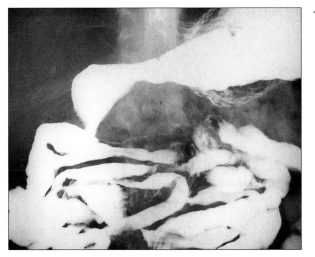

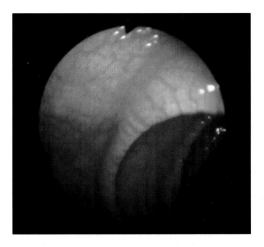

▲ **33, 34** A 46-year-old woman presented with iron deficiency and pale stools. The appearances on barium follow-through radiograph are very abnormal. An endoscopic view of the duodenal mucosa is shown in **34.**
(a) What abnormalities are shown on the radiograph?
(b) What abnormality is shown by endoscopy?
(c) What is the diagnosis and how is it confirmed?

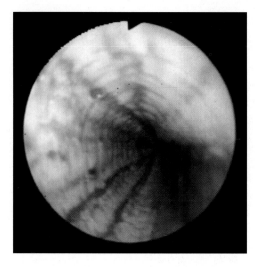

◀ **35** This endoscopic view of the oesophagus was taken from a patient who had attempted to commit suicide by ingesting cleaning solution containing sodium hydroxide. Give two possible late complications.

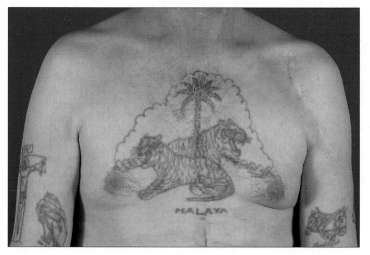

▲ **36** This man has cirrhosis.
(a) What cause for cirrhosis can be inferred from his appearance?
(b) What practical advice should be given to his family?

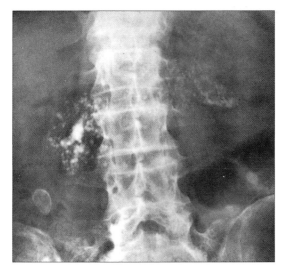

◀ **37** This plain abdominal radiograph was obtained from a man with chronic upper abdominal pain.
(a) What abnormality is shown?
(b) What is the diagnosis?

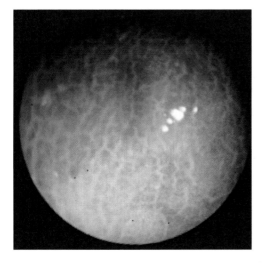

◀ **38** Colonoscopy revealed this appearance in a 56-year-old woman undergoing investigation for chronic diarrhoea.
(a) What abnormality is shown?
(b) How might this appearance be related to the cause of her diarrhoea?

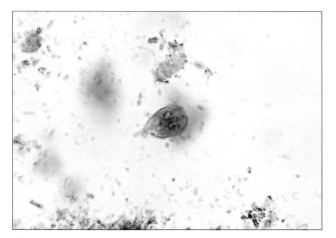

▲ **39** A 30-year-old man presented with a 3-week history of diarrhoea, upper abdominal cramps and weight loss. What abnormality is shown in this iron–haematoxylin wet stool preparation?

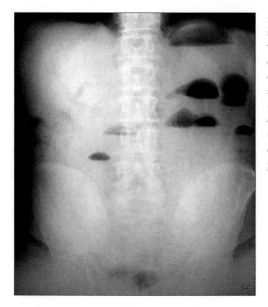

◀ **40** An erect plain abdominal radiograph was obtained from an elderly woman with colicky abdominal pain and vomiting.
(a) What features are demonstrated?
(b) What sequence of events has led to this presentation?

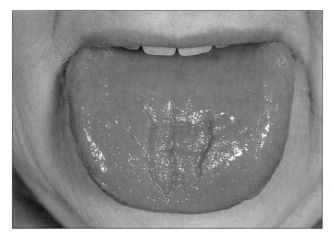

▲ **41** This shows the appearance of the tongue of a patient who presented with numbness and paraesthesiae of the feet. What is the cause of her neurological symptoms?

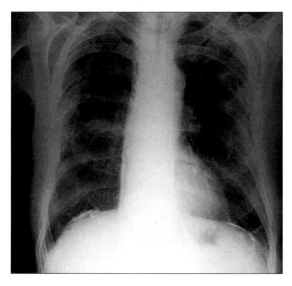

◀ **42** A 70-year-old man presented with ascites. The fluid was drained before further investigations were undertaken.
(a) What major abnormality is shown on his chest radiograph?
(b) How might this relate to the cause of his ascites?

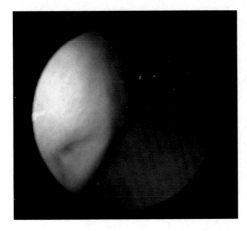

43 A 68-year-old woman underwent endoscopic investigation after two episodes of haematemesis and melaena within a month.
(a) What is the diagnosis?
(b) What rare complication may develop within these lesions?
(c) What treatment would you recommend?

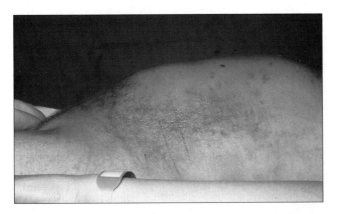

44 A 38-year-old woman who lived alone was found lying on the floor unconscious. She was markedly dehydrated, hypotensive and had a distended abdomen due to ascites. Bowel sounds were absent.
(a) What name is given to the physical sign seen here?
(b) What is the diagnosis?
(c) What has caused this appearance to develop?

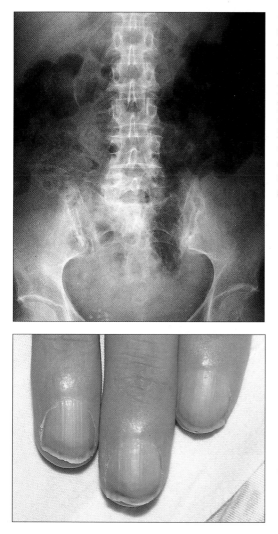

◄ **45** This plain abdominal radiograph was obtained from a 70-year-old woman with altered bowel habit during the past year.
(a) What abnormality is shown?
(b) What is the diagnosis?
(c) What is the standard treatment?

▲ **46** This photograph features the fingers of a 58-year-old man with a history of recent ankle swelling.
(a) What abnormality is shown?
(b) What biochemical abnormality is thought to account for this appearance?
(c) Give two possible diagnoses.

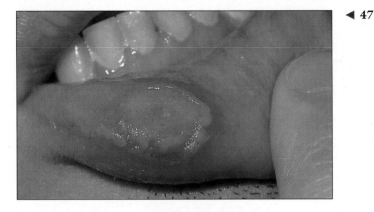

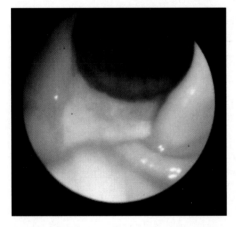

▲ **47, 48** A 37-year-old man developed painful mouth ulceration and rectal bleeding. The only abnormality on colonoscopy was a large rectal ulcer (**48**).
(a) What uncommon disorder do you suspect?
(b) Give three other features of this disorder.

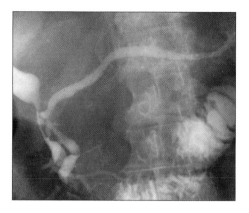

◀ **49** A 71-year-old woman gave a 3-week history of weight loss and obstructive jaundice. Ultrasound demonstrated a dilated biliary tree and several stones in the gall bladder. Endoscopic retrograde cholangiopancreatography (ERCP) was performed.
(a) What is the reason for her jaundice?
(b) Give two possible alternatives for treatment

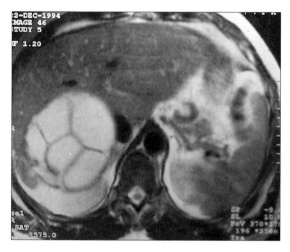

▲ **50** A 51-year-old farmer was referred with abdominal discomfort and an enlarged liver. Magnetic resonance imaging (MRI) was carried out.
(a) What is the diagnosis?
(b) What is the treatment of choice?

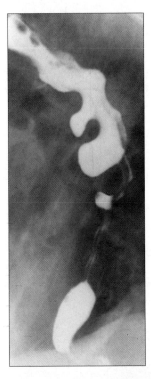

◀ **51** A barium swallow examination was done in a 78-year-old woman with dysphagia. What is the cause of her symptoms?

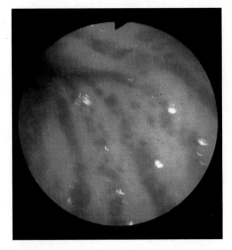

◀ **52** A 70-year-old woman was endoscoped because of recurrent iron-deficiency anaemia.
(a) What term is given to this characteristic appearance in the antrum of the stomach?
(b) Give two possible modes of treatment.

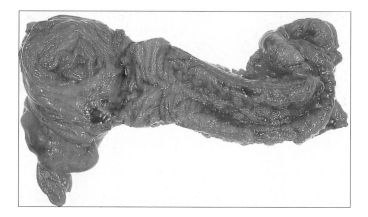

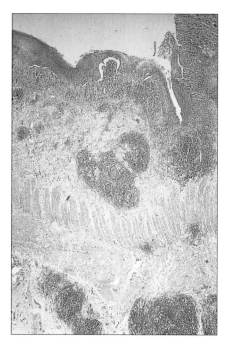

▲ 53, 54 This is a surgical resection specimen from a young woman with a long history of central colicky abdominal pain. A photomicrograph of the affected bowel is shown in **54**.

(a) Describe the abnormalities in the resection specimen.

(b) What is the diagnosis?

(c) Which three characteristic histological features of this disorder are shown in **54**?

◄ **54**

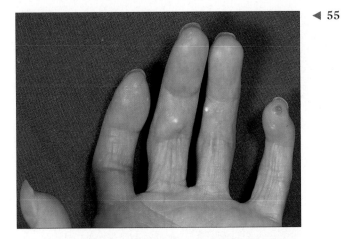

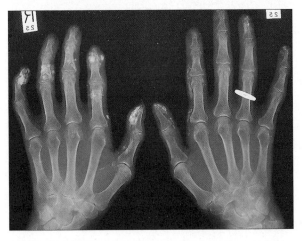

▲ **55, 56** (a) What three abnormalities are shown in this woman's hands?
(b) Which two other abnormalities are likely to coexist in this patient?

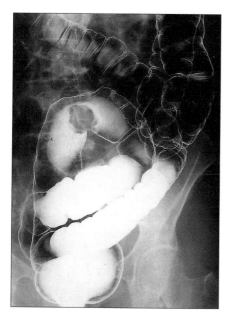

◀ **57** A barium enema examination was done to investigate rectal bleeding in a 67-year-old man.
(a) What abnormality is shown?
(b) Which further investigation should be done and why?
(c) What treatment would you recommend?

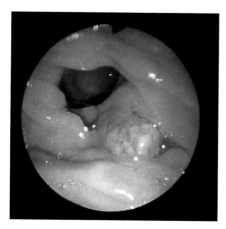

◀ **58** A 55-year-old man presented with a 3-week history of jaundice and dark urine.
(a) What two abnormalities are shown on duodenoscopy?
(b) What is the standard treatment?

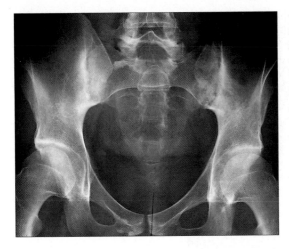

◀ **59** A 39-year-old man presented with a 2-month history of diarrhoea and rectal bleeding. Does this pelvic radiograph give you any clue as to the cause of his symptoms?

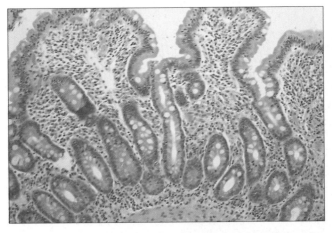

▲ **60** This section is from a small bowel biopsy taken from a female missionary with a 6-month history of diarrhoea and weight loss.
(a) What abnormality is shown?
(b) What is the likely diagnosis?
(c) What treatment would you recommend?

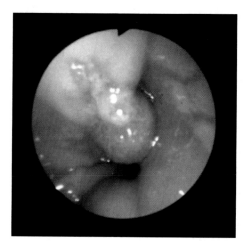

◄ **61** What abnormality is shown on endoscopy in this 23-year-old man with haematemesis?

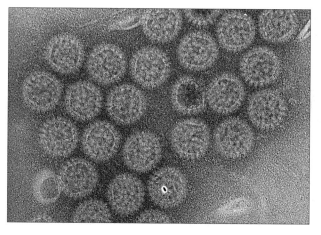

▲ **62** This electron micrograph was obtained from examination of the stool of an infant with sudden-onset diarhoea. What is the diagnosis?

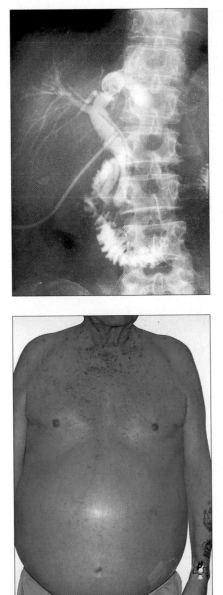

◀ **63** A 54-year-old man from Hong Kong presented with fever, jaundice and rigors. Cholecystectomy was performed, but no calculus could be found in the common bile duct. A T-tube was left *in situ* and this cholangiogram was performed 10 days postoperatively.

(a) What abnormalities are shown?

(b) What is the diagnosis?

(c) What late complication may develop?

◀ **64** (a) What three abnormalities are apparent?

(b) What is the diagnosis?

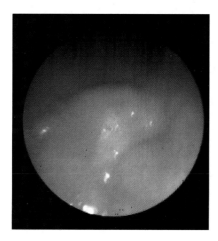

65 A 64-year-old man was endoscoped because of recent-onset dyspepsia. This lesion was found in the gastric antrum.
(a) What diagnosis would you suspect?
(b) What is the treatment?
(c) How does pathological examination help in evaluating the prognosis?

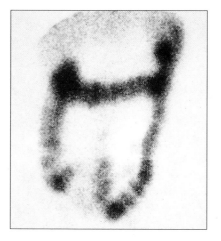

▲ 66 (a) What investigation has been performed?
(b) What is the diagnosis?

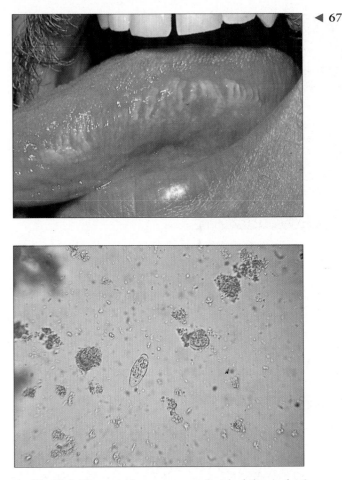

▲ **67, 68** A 28-year-old man presented with abdominal pain, diarrhoea and weight loss. He was an unmarried travelling salesman who regularly visited Africa. A smear of formol-ether stool concentrate is shown in **68**.
(a) What term is given to the tongue abnormality?
(b) What abnormality is shown in the stool?
(c) What is the underlying diagnosis?

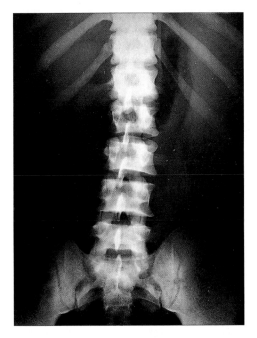

◀ **69** A 66-year-old man was sent for investigation of anaemia.
(a) Give two abnormalities on this plain abdominal radiograph.
(b) What is the diagnosis?

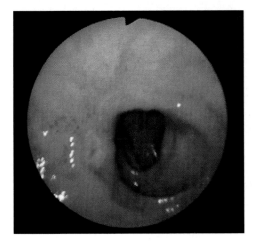

◀ **70** A 47-year-old man was endoscoped 3 days after having passed a melaena stool. He had been on no medication. An ulcer was found in the first part of the duodenum.
(a) Which two other important endoscopic features are shown?
(b) Give one further important investigation.
(c) Give two possible medical strategies for treatment.

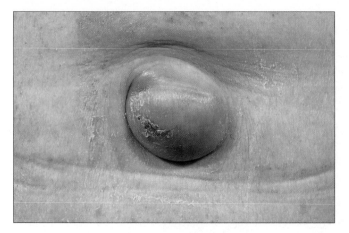

▲ 71 A 68-year-old woman receiving treatment for hepatic cirrhosis and ascites developed sudden onset central abdominal pain and faeculent vomiting. What abnormality of the umbilicus is shown and what complication has arisen?

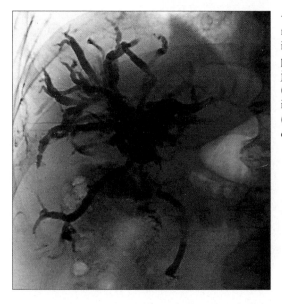

◀ 72 An 80-year-old man is being investigated for painless obstructive jaundice.
(a) What investigation is being performed?
(b) What is the likely diagnosis?

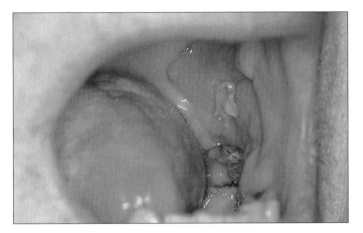

▲ **73** Biopsy of this oral lesion revealed multiple noncaseating granulomas. Give two possible diagnoses.

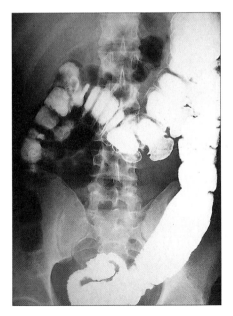

◄ **74** A 32-year-old man had experienced left iliac fossa pain and rectal bleeding for 2 months. Double contrast barium enema examination was performed but the patient had difficulty retaining the air and contrast. Therefore a single contrast study was carried out. (a) Describe the abnormalities. (b) What is the probable diagnosis?

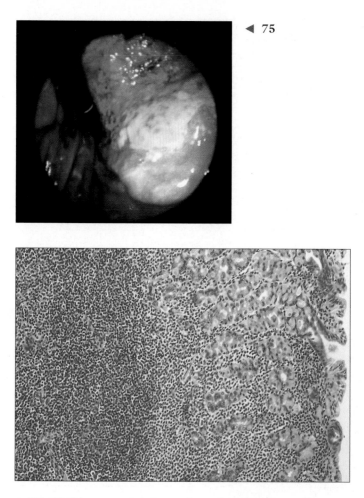

▲ **75, 76** Gastroscopy is being performed to investigate a 56-year-old man with upper abdominal pain and weight loss. **76** is a photomicrograph from a biopsy taken from this lesion.
(a) What is the diagnosis?
(b) What is the standard treatment?

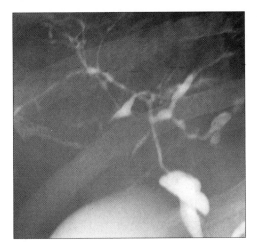

◀ **77** A 42-year-old man was referred with painless progressive jaundice and recurrent fever.
(a) What investigation is being performed?
(b) What is the diagnosis?
(c) Which associated gastrointestinal disease may also be present in this man?

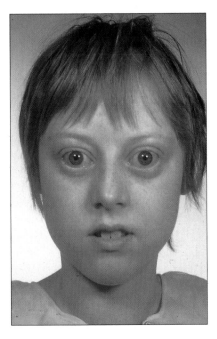

◀ **78** This young woman had been diagnosed as having an irritable bowel in another hospital and was referred for a second opinion. Her diarrhoea had become more troublesome and she had lost weight.
(a) What two abnormalities are apparent?
(b) What is the correct diagnosis?

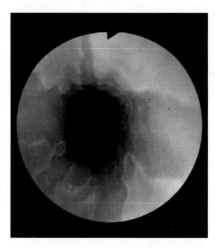

◀ **79** This photograph was taken with the tip of the endoscope positioned in the oesophagus 28 cm from the incisor teeth.
(a) What feature is demonstrated?
(b) What is the diagnosis?
(c) Give three late complications that may develop in this patient.

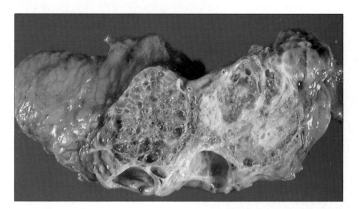

▲ **80** This lesion was found in the pancreas at autopsy. Give two possible diagnoses.

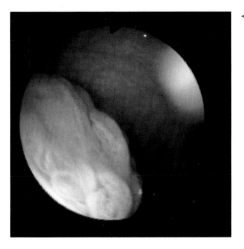

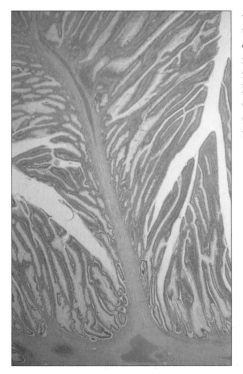

◀ **81, 82** An elderly man underwent investigations for diarrhoea. This lesion was found in the upper rectum on flexible sigmoidoscopy. The histology is shown in **82**.
(a) What is the diagnosis?
(b) Give two options for treatment.

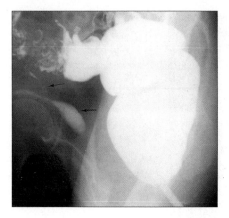

◀ **83** This lateral view of a barium enema radiograph shows a fistulous track between the sigmoid colon and bladder vault. Give three diseases that may lead to this complication.

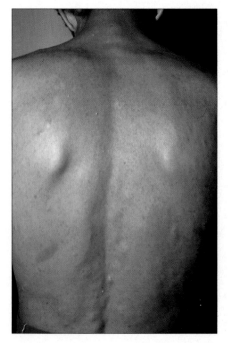

◀ **84** This man presented with frequent incontinence of faeces. What is the diagnosis and why does he have incontinence?

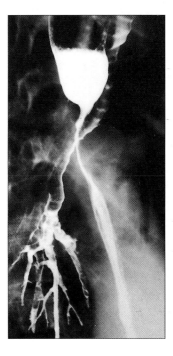

◀ **85** A 72-year-old man presented with dysphagia and a cough with purulent sputum. A barium swallow was performed.
(a) What is the most likely diagnosis?
(b) What complication has developed?
(c) How would the patient be best managed?

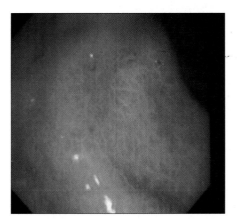

◀ **86** Gastroscopy is being performed to investigate anaemia in a patient with autoimmune (chronic active) hepatitis. What descriptive term is given for this gastric mucosal appearance?

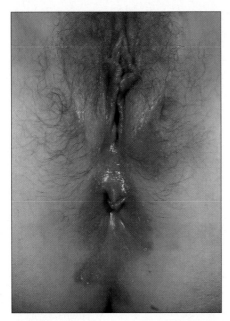

87 (a) What is the diagnosis? (b) What drug treatment would you recommend?

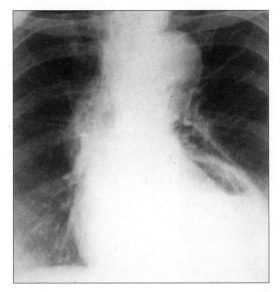

88 What abnormality is shown on this chest radiograph?

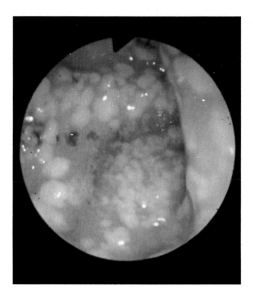

◀ **89** A 72-year-old woman on an intensive care unit was referred because of diarrhoea. She had required mechanical ventilation after severe pneumonia. This appearance was found on flexible sigmoidoscopy.
(a) What is the diagnosis?
(b) What is the treatment?
(c) What nursing precautions should be taken?

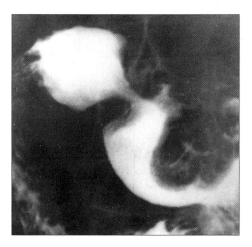

◀ **90** A 60-year-old man with recurrent profuse vomiting underwent a barium meal examination.
(a) What abnormality is shown?
(b) What metabolic abnormality could develop in this patient?

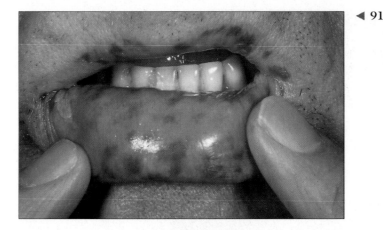

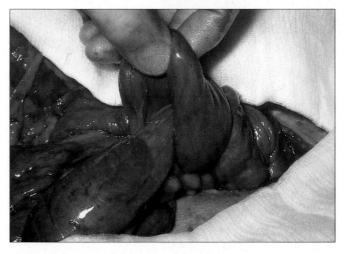

▲ **91, 92** A 28-year-old man developed sudden-onset central abdominal pain and vomiting. A photograph of the findings at laparotomy is shown in **92**.
(a) What is the diagnosis?
(b) What complication has occurred?
(c) Give two other complications of this disorder.

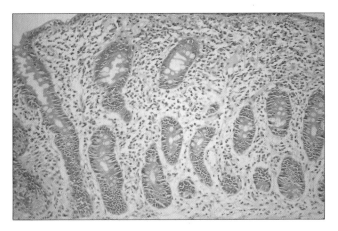

▲ **93** (a) What is the commonest cause of this appearance on small bowel biopsy?
(b) For which malignancies does this disorder confer an increased risk?

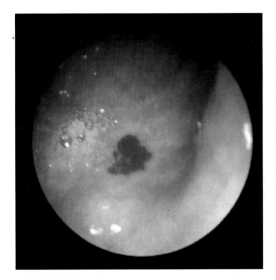

◀ **94** A 78-year-old man underwent upper gastrointestinal endoscopy for the investigation of iron–deficiency anaemia.
(a) What abnormality is shown in the first part of the duodenum?
b) How would you manage this patient?

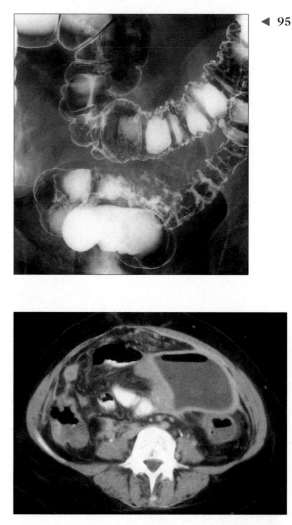

▲ **95, 96** A 34-year-old woman with Crohn's disease was admitted with a 2-week history of left iliac fossa pain.
(a) What abnormal features are visible on the barium enema radiograph in **95**?
(b) What complication is evident from the CT scan of the lower abdomen in **96**?
(c) Give two possible approaches to management.

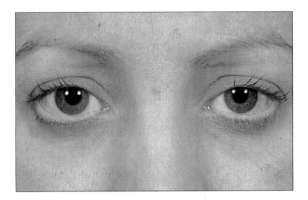

▲ **97** A 34-year-old woman had suffered severe epigastric pain for 24 h. Her father and sister had previously undergone splenectomy.
(a) What is the most likely diagnosis?
(b) How is this disorder inherited?
(c) What complication has developed?

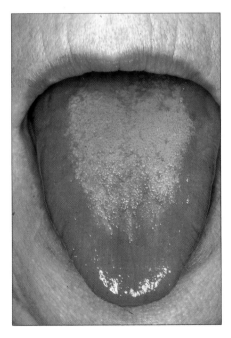

◀ **98** (a) What abnormality is evident on inspection?
(b) What is the likely underlying cause?

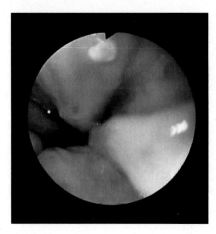

◄ **99** This is the appearance of the lower oesophagus of a 49-year-old man with recent haematemesis.
(a) What major abnormality is shown?
(b) There are two associated endoscopic features present that are associated with an increased bleeding risk. Can you name these?

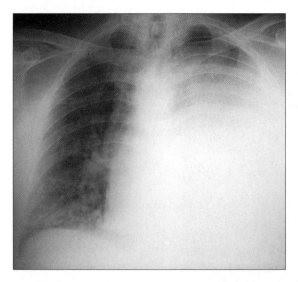

▲ **100** A 56-year-old man had been out for a large meal that had been accompanied by generous quantities of beer. He had woken at 3 a.m. with profuse vomiting, followed by severe central chest and back pain.
(a) What abnormalities are seen on his chest radiograph?
(b) What has caused his pain and the radiograph changes?

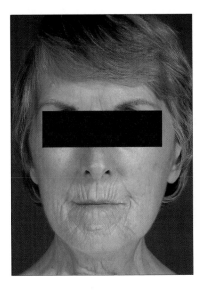

◀ **101** This woman presented with steatorrhoea. How might this have arisen?

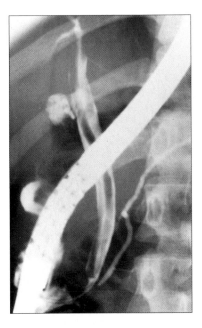

◀ **102** (a) What abnormality has been shown by ERCP?
(b) Give two approaches to treatment.

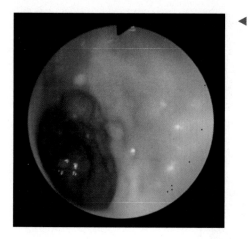

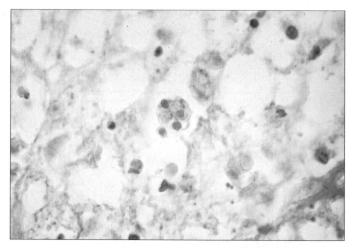

▲ **103, 104** A colonoscopic view from a 32-year-old man with a 4-week history of diarrhoea and rectal bleeding. He had recently returned from Uganda. Stool cultures were negative. Part of a biopsy specimen is shown in **104.**

(a) What is the diagnosis?

(b) What treatment would you advise?

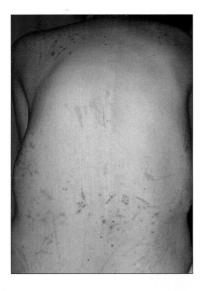

◀ **105** This photograph was taken from a patient with recently diagnosed schizophrenia who had become slightly jaundiced.
(a) What abnormality is shown?
(b) What is the diagnosis?
(c) How would you manage this patient?

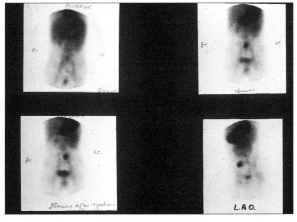

▲ **106** A 22-year-old woman is being investigated for repeated episodes of dark–red rectal bleeding. Sequential images have been taken after intravenous injection of ^{99}Technetium pertechnetate. What abnormality is shown?

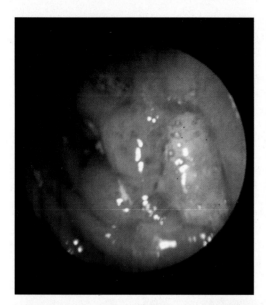

◀ **107** This endoscopic view is of an ulcer arising from the posterior body of the stomach in a 36-year-old man. It had failed to heal despite 3 months of omeprazole therapy.

(a) Give three possible reasons why the ulcer has not healed.

(b) Give two relevant further investigations.

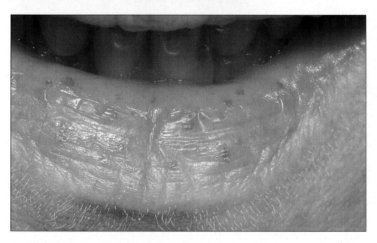

▲ **108** (a) What abnormality is seen?

(b) What is the diagnosis?

(c) Give two possible presenting manifestations.

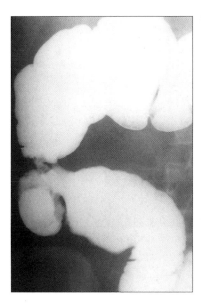

◀ **109, 110** A 62-year-old chef gave a 3-month history of fever, colicky central abdominal pain and weight loss. On examination there was a tender mass palpable in the right iliac fossa. The appearances on barium enema examination are shown in **109**. Right hemicolectomy was performed. A photomicrograph of part of the intestinal submucosa is shown in **110**.
(a) What is the diagnosis?
(b) Which characteristic histological feature is seen in **110**?

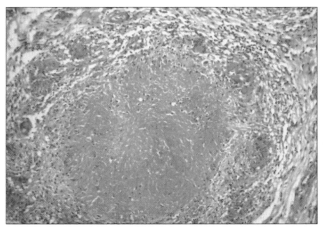

◀ **110**

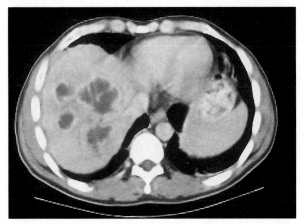

▲ 111 A 56-year-old man with Crohn's disease developed
fever without any other symptoms of disease relapse. This
appearance was obtained by CT scan after intravenous
injection of contrast.
(a) What is the diagnosis?
(b) What treatment would you recommend?

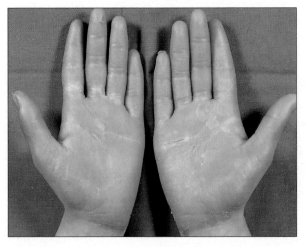

▲ 112 This skin disorder has been reported to occur rarely
in an inherited form associated with oesophageal cancer. Can
you name the skin disorder?

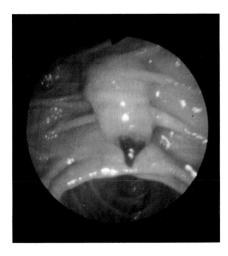

◄ **113, 114** A 36-year-old man was admitted for investigation of abnormal liver function tests. Upper abdominal ultrasound was normal. Percutaneous liver biopsy followed by endoscopic retrograde cholangiography was performed. The appearance of the ampulla of Vater before cholangiography is shown in **113**, and **114** demonstrates the cholangiographic appearances.
(a) What phenomenon has been demonstrated?
(b) What had precipitated this phenomenon?

◄ **114**

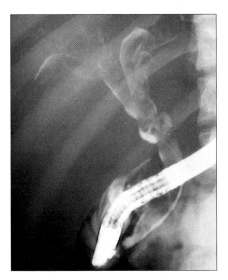

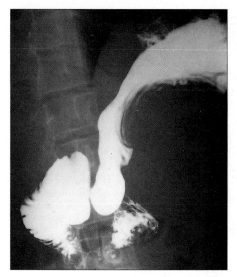

◄ **115** A 42-year-old man had suffered from epigastric pain for 3 weeks.
(a) What abnormality is demonstrated on this barium meal radiograph?
(b) What is the diagnosis and how would you confirm it?
(c) What treatment is recommended?

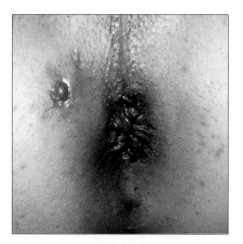

▲ **116** (a) What abnormality is shown?
(b) Give two possible predisposing factors.

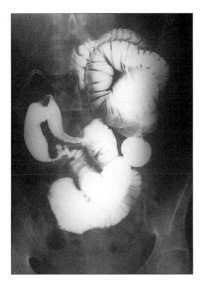

117 A 42-year-old woman is being investigated for colicky abdominal pain and weight loss.
(a) What investigation is being performed?
(b) What abnormalities are shown?
(c) What is the likely diagnosis?

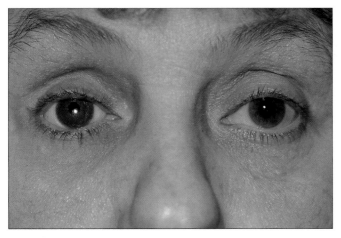

▲ **118** How might this woman's appearance be related to her hepatic enlargement and tenderness?

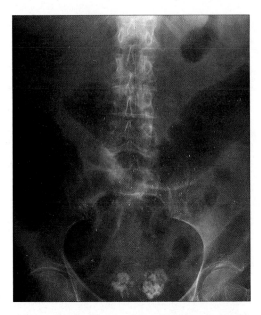

◀ **119** This patient had suffered copious diarrhoea for 3 weeks.
(a) What does this plain abdominal radiograph show?
(b) Which disease most commonly gives rise to this appearance?
(c) Give two other diseases that can cause this phenomenon.

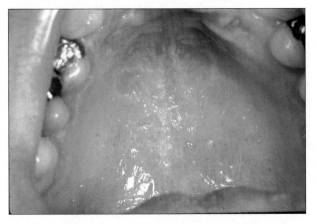

▲ **120** A 22-year-old man developed a maculopapular rash, generalised lymphadenopathy and mild fever. Liver function tests showed marked elevation of plasma alkaline phosphatase. Inspection of the hard palate revealed ulceration, which had been painless.
(a) What is the diagnosis?
(b) How is this confirmed?

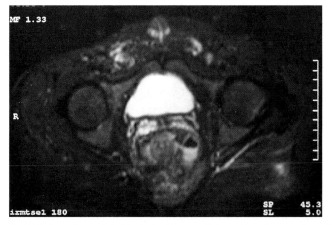

▲ **121** A patient with Crohn's disease of the colon, but sparing the rectum, underwent MRI to investigate severe left iliac fossa pain and fever. What abnormality is demonstrated?

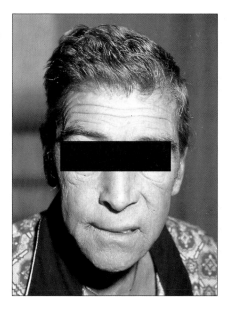

◀ **122** This man had recently developed diabetes mellitus. There was no history of alcohol excess. Examination of the abdomen revealed an enlarged liver, which was smooth and non tender.
(a) What is the diagnosis?
(b) What is the treatment?
(c) Which important late complication is not prevented by this treatment?

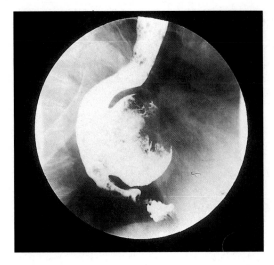

123 An 88-year-old woman underwent a barium swallow examination to investigate intermittent regurgitation after food. What abnormality is demonstrated?

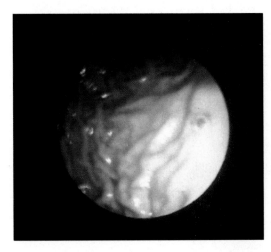

124 A 78-year-old woman underwent gastroscopy the day after a large haematemesis with melaena stool. The cause for bleeding is seen here high up on the lesser curvature and posterior body of the stomach.
(a) What abnormality is shown?
(b) How should this be treated?

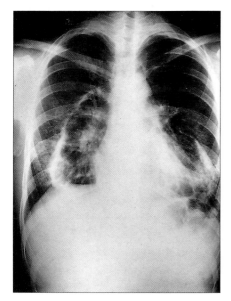

125 A 64-year-old man had been diagnosed with ulcerative colitis 1 year before. He remained in remission while taking sulphasalazine. He had become breathless during the past 2 weeks. This is his chest radiograph.
(a) What has caused this appearance?
(b) How should he be managed?

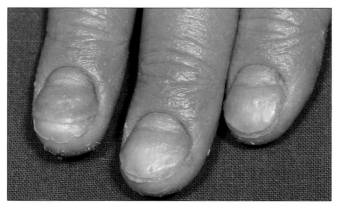

▲ 126 A 46-year-old man was transferred from the dermatology ward because he had recently developed ascites.
(a) What has caused these nail changes?
(b) Which preventable complication may have caused his ascites?

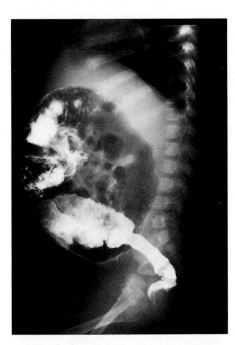

◀ **127** This is a lateral barium enema radiograph from an infant presenting with abdominal distension.
(a) What features are shown?
(b) What is the diagnosis?

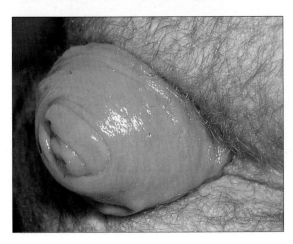

◀ **128** This photograph is from a 67-year-old man who complained of faecal incontinence.
(a) What abnormality is shown?
(b) What treatment would you suggest?

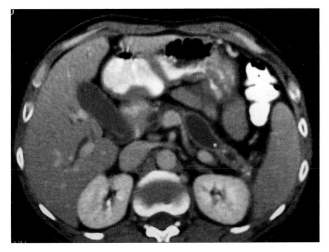

▲ 129 A CT scan was done to investigate a 38-year-old man with recurrent epigastric pain radiating to the back.
(a) What abnormalities are shown?
(b) What is the diagnosis?
(c) What is the most likely predisposing factor?

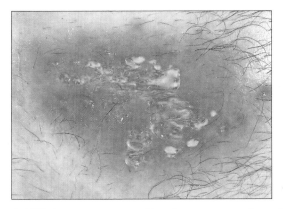

▲ 130 A young man attending the gastroenterology clinic presented with this lesion on his forearm.
(a) What is the lesion?
(b) What is the associated gastroenterological disease?
(c) How would the skin lesion be treated?

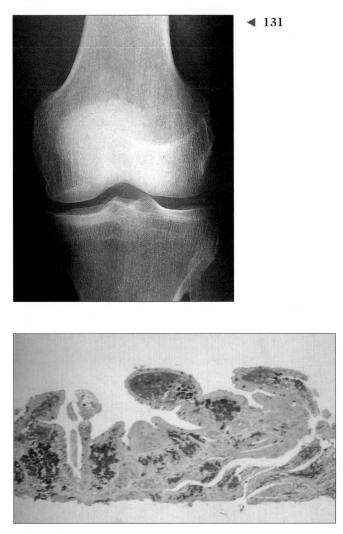

▲ **131, 132** A 64-year-old man presented with arthritis of both knees. He was found to be anaemic with low serum calcium. He underwent jejunal biopsy. The photomicrograph in **132** has been stained using the PAS technique.

(a) What abnormality is shown on the radiograph?

(b) What is the diagnosis?

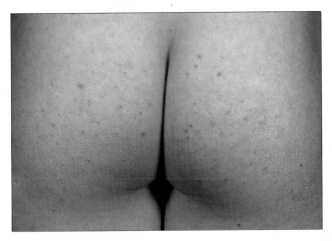

▲ 133 A 14-year-old boy developed abdominal pain and a papular rash.
(a) What is the diagnosis?
(b) Give two potentially serious complications of this disorder.

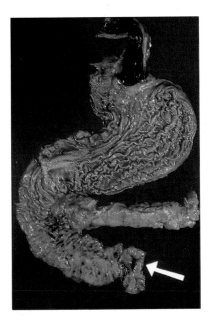

◄ 134 This slide was taken at autopsy. There was a tumour in the head of the pancreas and there were multiple perforations of the third part of the duodenum. Can you explain these findings?

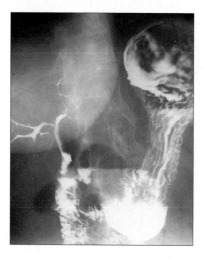

◀ **135** A 65-year-old woman presented with fever, rigors and dark urine.

(a) What is the most likely cause of this appearance on the barium meal radiograph?

(b) What complication has developed?

(c) Give two possible explanations as to how this complication may have developed.

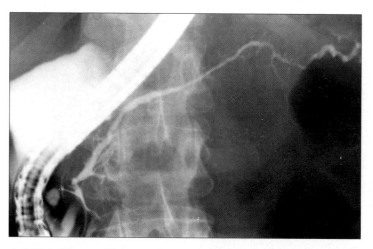

▲ **136** A 52-year-old man underwent investigation for chronic upper abdominal pain.

(a) What abnormality is shown on this ERCP?

(b) What is the diagnosis?

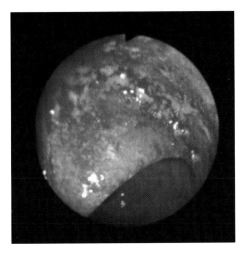

◀ **137, 138** A 40-year-old man gave a 2-week history of bloodstained diarrhoea. Stool cultures were negative. The appearance of the upper rectal mucosa is shown in **137**. A photomicrograph of a rectal biopsy specimen can be seen in **138**.
(a) What endoscopic features are shown?
(b) What is the diagnosis?
(c) How does the biopsy help in predicting the future course of the illness?

◀ **138**

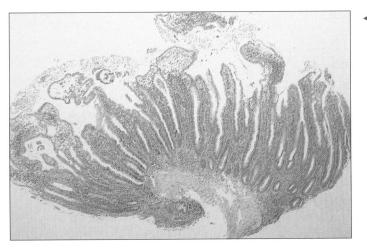

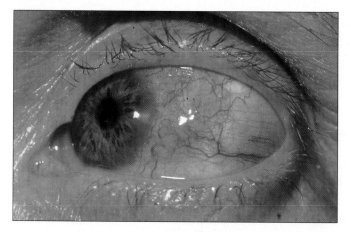

▲ **139** (a) What abnormality is shown?
(b) With which gastroenterological disorder may this be associated?

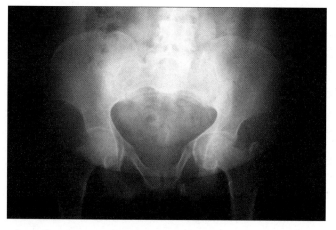

▲ **140** (a) What is the major abnormality?
(b) What disorder underlies this radiograph appearance?
(c) Give three possible causes of this disorder.

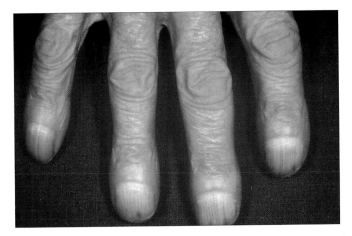

▲ **141** Give five gastroenterological associations.

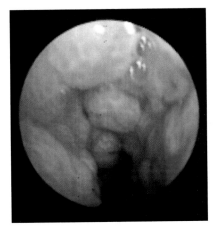

◄ **142** A 66-year-old man presented with weight loss and epigastric discomfort. At endoscopy the stomach would not distend properly in response to air insufflation.
(a) What term is given to this endoscopic appearance?
(b) What is the diagnosis?

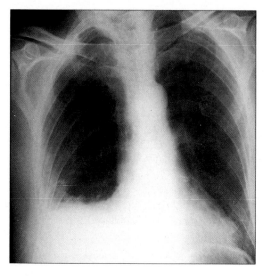

▲ **143** A 72-year-old man had been taking non-steroidal anti-inflammatory drugs for osteoarthritis. He presented with a 1-week long history of pyrexia, right upper quadrant pain and weight loss.
(a) What abnormality is shown on the chest radiograph?
(b) What is the likely diagnosis?

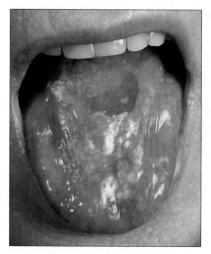

◀ **144** A 56-year-old woman presented with dysphagia. On examination there was a papular purplish eruption over the wrists and forearms. The tongue is also affected by this disorder.
(a) What is the diagnosis?
(b) What oesophageal manifestations of this disorder are recognised?
(c) What treatment should be considered?

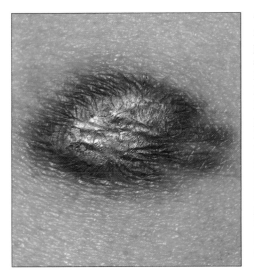

◄ **145, 146** A 30-year-old man presented with profound weight loss and supraclavicular lymphadenopathy. This lesion was noted on the lateral chest wall. A photomicrograph of a lymph node biopsy stained by the Ziehl-Neelsen method is shown in **146**.
(a) What is the skin lesion?
(b) What striking feature is present on lymph node biopsy?
(c) What is the underlying diagnosis?

◄ **146**

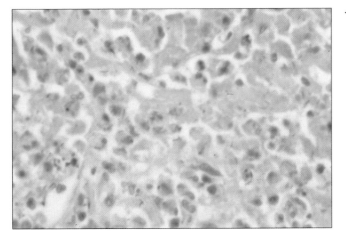

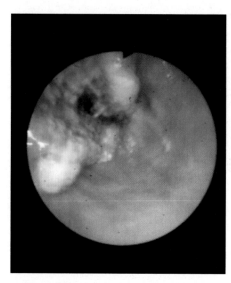

◄ 147, 148 An 82-year-old
man presented with dysphagia.
This photograph was taken
with the tip of the endoscope
25 cm below the incisor teeth.
A photomicrograph of a biopsy
from the lesion can be seen in
148.
(a) What is the diagnosis?
(b) What non-surgical
treatments are available?

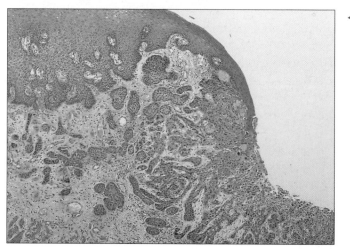

◄ 148

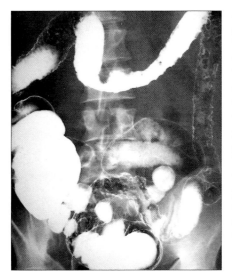

149 A 32-year-old man with a 2-month history of bloodstained diarrhoea and weight loss was referred because his presumed ulcerative colitis had not improved on twice-daily steroid enemas. He was heterosexual and stool microscopy and culture showed no pathogens. An 'instant' barium enema was performed without prior bowel preparation.
(a) Describe the abnormalities on the radiograph.
(b) Why is the rectum spared?

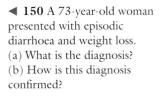

150 A 73-year-old woman presented with episodic diarrhoea and weight loss.
(a) What is the diagnosis?
(b) How is this diagnosis confirmed?

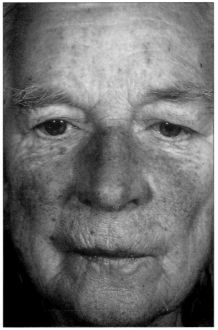

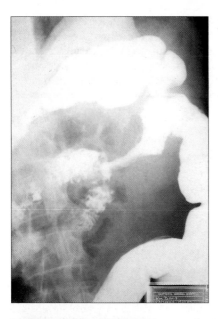

◀ **151** A 62-year-old man underwent barium enema examination to investigate the abrupt onset of diarrhoea and loss of 5 kg in weight.
(a) What abnormality is demonstrated?
(b) What is the most likely underlying cause?
(c) Why has diarrhoea developed?

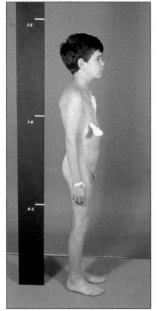

◀ **152** A 16-year-old boy was referred for investigation of short stature, lack of pubertal development and recent proximal muscle weakness. He was found to be anaemic, and three stool samples were positive for occult blood.
(a) Which gastrointestinal disorder should be considered?
(b) Give three possible ways of confirming the diagnosis.

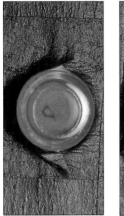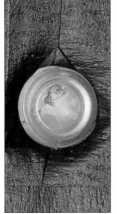

◀ **153** A test is commercially available for the examination of gastric biopsy tissue. Antral biopsies from two patients were obtained and one placed in the left-hand vial and the other in the right-hand one. Photographs were taken 2 h after the biopsies were placed in their respective media.
(a) What kind of test is this?
(b) What does this tell us about these two patients?
(c) What are the main indications for performing this test?

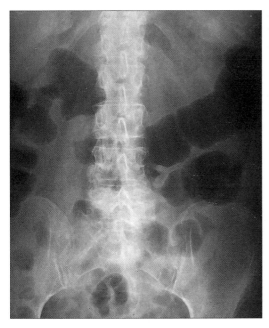

◀ **154** A 73-year-old woman presented with sudden onset central abdominal pain and bloodstained diarrhoea.
(a) What abnormality is seen on the plain abdominal radiograph?
(b) What is the diagnosis?
(c) What late complication may develop?

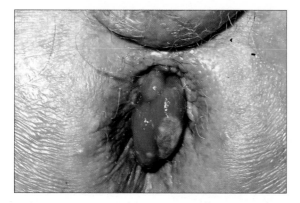

▲ **155** A 68-year-old man complained of pruritus ani and discharge.
(a) What abnormality is shown?
(b) What is the treatment of choice?

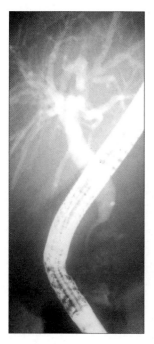

◀ **156** This endoscopic retrograde cholangiogram was performed in a 56-year-old man with a 10-year history of recurrent epigastric pain and recent jaundice.
(a) What abnormalities are seen?
(b) What is the diagnosis?

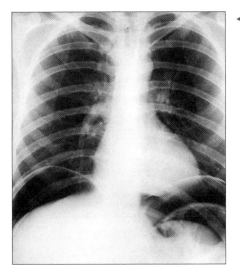

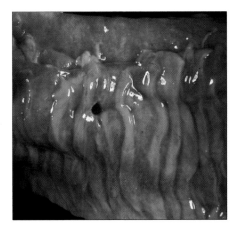

▲ **157, 158** An 82-year-old man with rheumatoid arthritis gave a 2-day history of abdominal pain. His chest radiograph on admission is shown in **157**, and **158** shows part of the jejunal resection specimen.
(a) What is the diagnosis?
(b) Give the most likely aetiological factor.

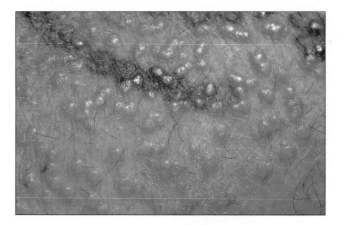

▲ 159 These lesions developed on the forearms of a 36-year-old man, who also gave a history of four previous hospital admissions because of acute abdominal pain.
(a) What are the lesions?
(b) What is the most likely underlying disorder?
(c) How do you explain the abdominal pain?

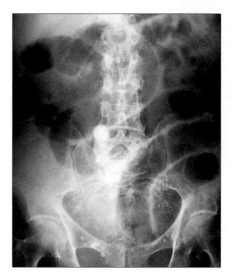

◄ 160 A 76-year-old woman had suffered severe colicky abdominal pain and faeculent vomiting for 18 h. The diagnosis and its underlying cause can be inferred from this plain abdominal radiograph.

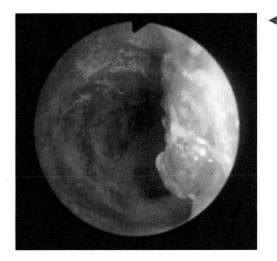

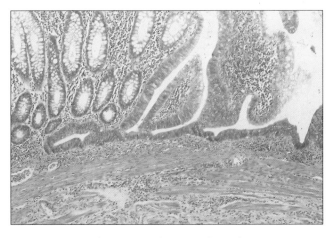

▲ **161, 162** A colonoscopy is being performed in a patient with a 25-year history of extensive ulcerative colitis. A biopsy from the lesion shown in **161** can be seen in **162**.

(a) What does the biopsy show?

(b) What complication has developed?

(c) What treatment would you recommend?

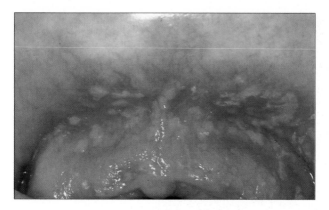

▲ **163** This rare pustular eruption of the buccal mucosa is strongly associated with inflammatory bowel disease. Can you name this disorder?

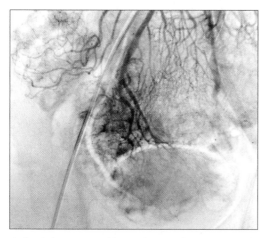

▲ **164** A 76-year-old man had undergone aortic valve replacement 6 years previously and had been on warfarin. He had been admitted several times since with dark–red rectal bleeding.
(a) What investigation is being performed?
(b) What is the diagnosis?

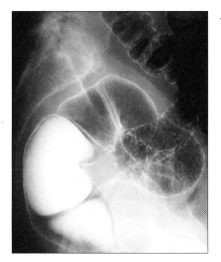

▲ 165, 166 A 50-year-old exporter presented with rectal bleeding; 165 is a lateral view of the rectosigmoid mucosa. A rectal biopsy was smeared on a glass slide and the unstained microscopic appearance is shown in 166.
(a) What is the diagnosis?
(b) What is the most common late complication of this disease?

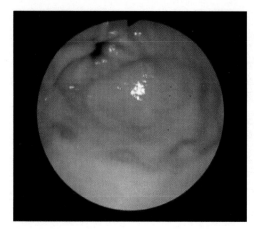

◀ **167** This view was obtained at the prepyloric region during gastroscopy of a patient who had passed a melaena stool 1 week previously. Past history included transient cerebral ischaemia.
(a) What abnormality is shown?
(b) What is the most likely cause of this lesion?

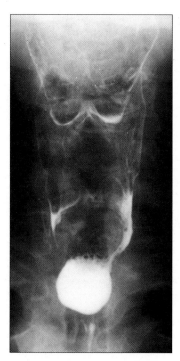

◀ **168** A barium swallow was performed to investigate regurgitation after meals in a 69-year-old woman.
(a) What abnormality is seen?
(b) What important late complication may occur?
(c) Should endoscopy be performed?
(d) How should she be managed?

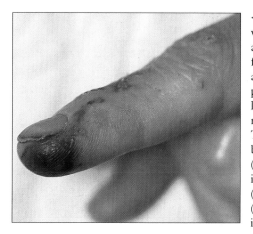

◀ **169, 170** A 72-year-old woman developed abdominal pain and fever. A few days later this lesion appeared on one digit. Her pain failed to resolve and laparotomy with small bowel resection was performed. The histology of the resected bowel is shown in **170**.
(a) What abnormality is seen in the photomicrograph?
(b) What is the diagnosis?
(c) Which serological investigation might support this diagnosis?

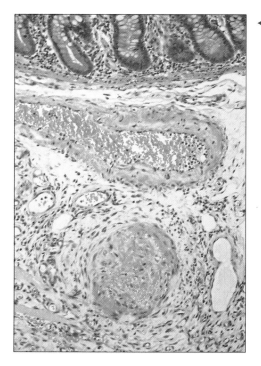

◀ **170**

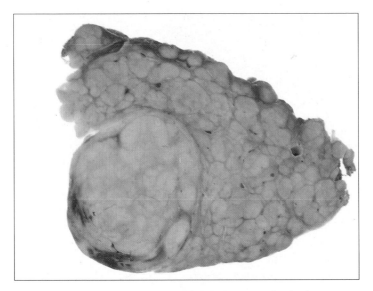

▲ **171** (a) Which two disease processes can be seen in this hepatic resection specimen?
(b) What is the most likely underlying cause?

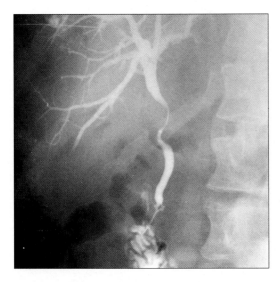

◀ **172** A 69-year-old man with no previous illness presented with jaundice and dark urine.
(a) What investigation is being performed?
(b) Give three possible diagnoses.

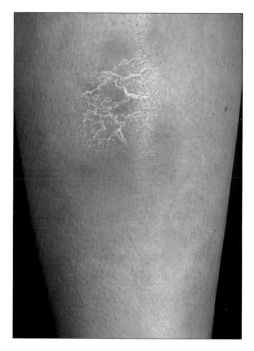

◀ **173, 174** A 30-year-old woman developed bloodstained diarrhoea and a painful swelling of her right leg. Proctoscopy showed no abnormality.
(a) What skin lesion is shown?
(b) Give three features shown by colonoscopy in **174**.
(c) What is the likely underlying diagnosis?

◀ **174**

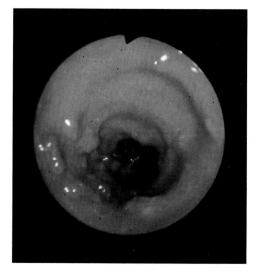

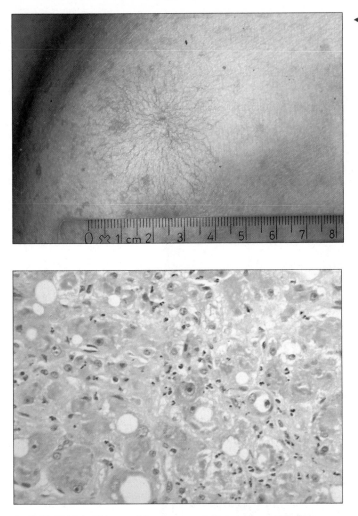

▲ **175, 176** A 60-year-old man was admitted after a fall. He was noted to be jaundiced and to have several capillary lesions. A liver biopsy was performed.
(a) What is the skin lesion?
(b) What abnormalities can you see on the biopsy shown in **176**?
(c) What is the diagnosis?

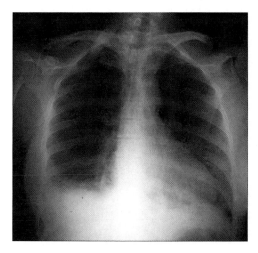

◀ **177** A 50-year-old woman presented with dysphagia. Endoscopy identified a tight stricture in the mid–oesophagus that could only just be negotiated with the tip of the scope. Multiple biopsies were taken. She developed chest pain the evening after the procedure.

(a) What is the major abnormality on the chest radiograph?

(b) How should she be managed?

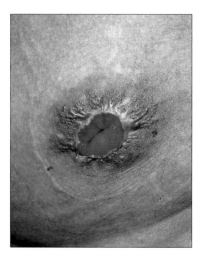

◀ **178** A 56-year-old man had undergone panproctocolectomy and ileostomy for ulcerative colitis 5 years previously. He complained of recurrent haemorrhage from around the stoma site.

(a) What is the cause of the recurrent haemorrhage?

(b) What is the most likely explanation for this phenomenon?

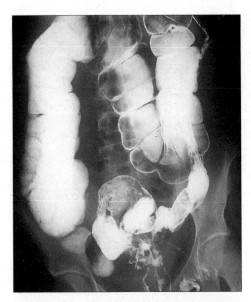

179 A 63-year-old man developed fever, constipation and pain in the left buttock.
(a) What abnormality is shown on his barium enema radioraph?
(b) How should he be managed?

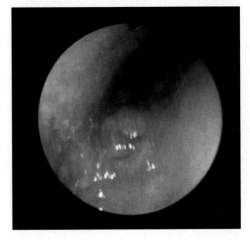

180 An elderly man with long–standing heartburn underwent oesophagoscopy for the investigation of anaemia. This photograph was taken with the tip of the endoscope positioned 30 cm below the incisor teeth. Give two macroscopic abnormalities.

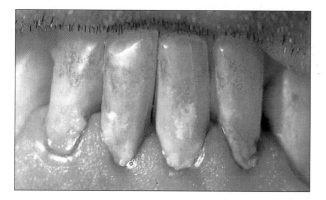

▲ **181** A 36-year-old man presented with colicky abdominal pain. As part of his job he dismantled car batteries.
(a) What abnormality is shown in the mouth?
(b) What is the diagnosis?

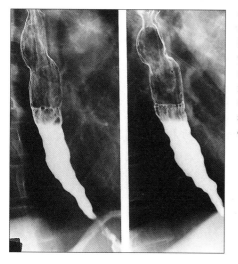

◄ **182** A barium swallow was done to investigate intermittent dysphagia in a 64-year-old man.
(a) Give three radiological features of note.
(b) What two investigations are done to confirm the diagnosis?

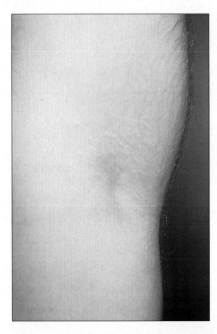

183 A 35-year-old woman presented with haematemesis and melaena. Her elbow flexures had an unusual appearance.

(a) What is the diagnosis?

(b) Where else, apart from the skin, would you look for signs of this disorder?

(c) Why does gastrointestinal haemorrhage develop in this condition?

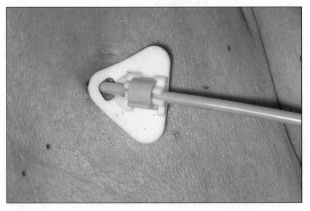

184 This patient requires enteral feeding by means of a percutaneous endoscopic gastrostomy. What are the two major indications for the use of these tubes?

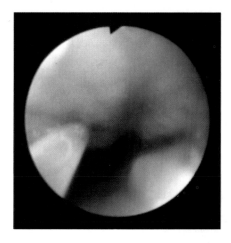

◀ **185** (a) What endoscopic treatment is being given for this patient with oesophageal varices?
(b) Give three possible complications of this technique.
(c) What alternative endoscopic treatment is available?

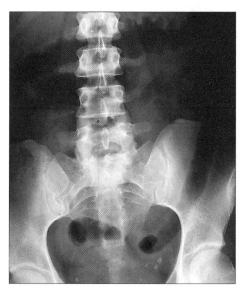

▲ **186** A 35-year-old woman presented with a 2-week history of bloodstained diarrhoea.
(a) Describe the abnormalities on this plain abdominal radiograph.
(b) What is the diagnosis?

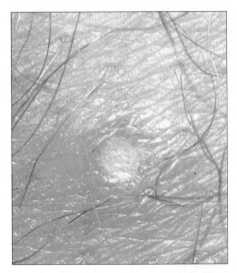

◀ **187** A 50-year-old man presented with melaena and shock. Several of these lesions were noted on the limbs and trunk.
(a) What is the diagnosis?
(b) What other gastrointestinal complication may occur?

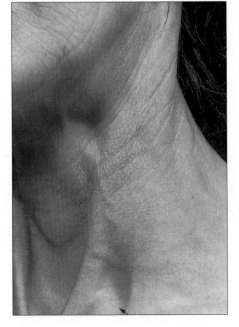

◀ **188** A 60-year-old woman had lost 8 kg over 3 months. She was found to have a haemoglobin concentration of 8 g/dl and a hypochromic microcytic blood film.
(a) What abnormality is shown?
(b) What is the probable underlying diagnosis?

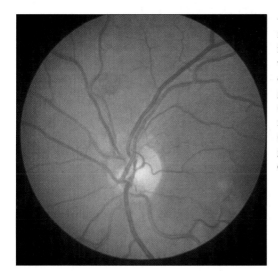

◀ **189** Fundoscopy revealed this appearance in a 20-year-old man with an inherited disorder affecting the gut.
(a) What abnormality is noted?
(b) What is the gastrointestinal diagnosis?

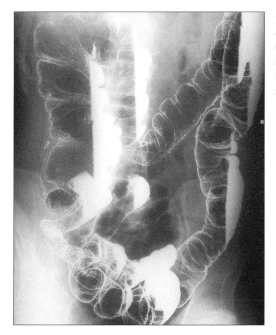

◀ **190** (a) What abnormalities are seen on this barium enema radiograph?
(b) What is the most likely diagnosis?

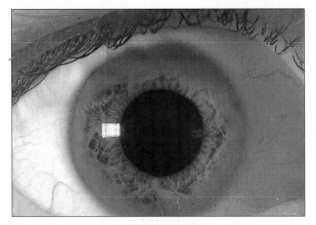

▲ 191 (a) What abnormality is seen?
(b) What is the diagnosis?
(c) Give three possible presenting manifestations of this condition.

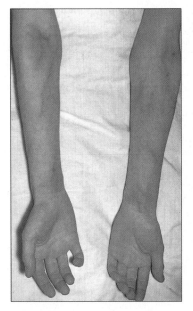

◄ 192 For which forms of viral hepatitis would this patient be at risk?

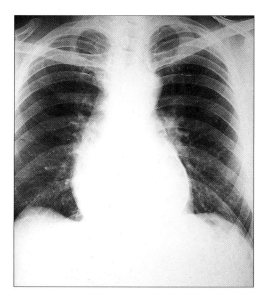

◄**193** A 51-year-old man presented with gross ascites and oedema.
(a) What abnormality is shown on his chest radiograph?
(b) What is the diagnosis?

ANSWERS

1, 2 (a) Candidiasis. The white plaques are characteristic. The photomicrograph is stained with PAS and the dark red branched fungal hyphae appear at top left of photograph.
(b) Diabetes mellitus, recent broad–spectrum antibiotic use, immunosuppression (e.g. AIDS, haematological malignancy, steroid therapy).

3 (a) Dermatitis herpetiformis.
(b) Biopsy and demonstration of granular IgA deposits in dermal papillae.
(c) Coeliac disease.

4 (a) Ménétrièr's disease (giant rugal hypertrophy).
(b) Protein loss through the gastric mucosa, leading to hypoalbuminaemia.

5 (a) Pigmentation, jaundice, xanthelasmata.
(b) Primary biliary cirrhosis.
(c) Referral for liver transplantation.

6 This man had been taking aspirin. All non-steroidal anti-inflammatory drugs can be associated with ulcers of the stomach, duodenum and small intestine. Slow-release potassium supplements have also been linked with non-specific ulcers. Another possible cause is gastric acid hypersecretion secondary to a gastrinoma (Zollinger-Ellison syndrome).

7 (a) Diverticulosis of the small intestine.
(b) Haemorrhage, perforation, malabsorption secondary to bacterial overgrowth (blind loop syndrome).

8 (a) Endoscopic retrograde cholangio-pancreatography (ERCP).
(b) Pancreatitis, cholangitis and, very rarely, duodenal perforation. All are more common after therapeutic manoeuvres such as sphincterotomy.

9, 10 (a) Iron deficiency - the nails are flattened, almost spoon-shaped (koilonychia) and the nail beds are pale.
(b) An oesophageal web is seen in the postcricoid region. The link between these webs and iron deficiency is termed the Plummer-Vinson or Paterson-Kelly syndrome.
(c) Postcricoid carcinoma.

11 (a) Perianal warts (condyloma acuminata).
(b) Human papilloma virus.

12 (a) Carcinoma of the colon.
(b) In the absence of polyps elsewhere in the colon this man may have hereditary non-polyposis colorectal cancer (HNPCC). A careful family history must be taken.

13   (a) Addison's disease (primary adrenal insufficiency) with buccal pigmentation.
(b) Short Synacthen test.

14   (a) Space-occupying lesion in right lobe with hypodense surrounding halo effect.
(b) Amoebic liver abscess.
(c) Amoebic serology, stool microscopy.
(d) Oral metronidazole or tinidazole. Aspiration may be required in larger abscesses
or if pyogenic abscess is possible.

15   Radiation-induced colonic stricture secondary to previous radiotherapy.

16   (a) Barium enema examination.
(b) Loss of haustral folds, granular mucosal surface.
(c) Ulcerative colitis.

17   (a) Acanthosis nigricans.
(b) Malignancy of stomach or pancreas.

18   (a) Benign oesophageal stricture with oesophagitis above.
(b) Healing of the oesophagitis with a proton pump inhibitor (e.g. omeprazole or
lansoprazole) will normally lead to reduction of dysphagia. Endoscopic dilatation
is occasionally necessary.

19, 20
(a) Acquired immune deficiency syndrome (AIDS) presenting in this way is termed
'slim disease'.
(b) Cryptosporidiosis (a few red-staining round coccidian parasites lie on the
epithelial surface).

21, 22
(a) Rheumatoid arthritis.
(b) Involvement of the gut by amyloidosis. Subepithelial eosinophilic (red–staining)
amyloid deposits are seen.

23   (a) Crohn's disease of the terminal ileum.
(b) Ileal tuberculosis, lymphoma.

24   Gastric varices.

25   (a) Diverticular disease of the colon.
(b) Carcinoma of the colon. It is impossible to exclude a carcinoma of the sigmoid
colon on this examination. The many overlapping loops of bowel make diagnosis
difficult and flexible sigmoidoscopy (or colonoscopy) is necessary.

26   (a) Macronodular cirrhosis.

(b) Autoimmune (chronic active) hepatitis, chronic hepatitis B, chronic hepatitis C.

27　(a) Scurvy. The gingival papillae are swollen and fragile.
(b) Inspection of limbs for purpura, hair follicles for perifollicular haemorrhages and hyperkeratosis.
(c) Measurement of leucocyte ascorbic acid concentration.

28　(a) Para-oesophageal (rolling) hiatus hernia.
(b) Surgical repair.

29　Threadworm (*Enterobius vermicularis*).

30　(a) *Helicobacter pylori*.
(b) Chronic superficial (Type B) gastritis, peptic ulcer, gastric carcinoma, gastric lymphoma (arising from mucosa-associated lymphoid tissue).

31　(a) Bilateral parotid gland enlargement.
(b) Alcoholic liver disease.

32　(a) Barium has entered the colon, which is shortened and ulcerated. The haustral pattern is lost. There is a cobbled appearance to the colonic mucosa.
(b) Crohn's disease of the colon.

33, 34
(a) Flocculation of barium and featureless jejunal mucosa. Comparison can be made with the more normal small intestinal mucosal pattern in the centre of **32.**
(b) The duodenal folds have accentuated furrows giving a 'scalloped' appearance.
(c) Coeliac disease (gluten–sensitive enteropathy) confirmed on duodenal or jejunal biopsy and subsequent clinical and histological improvement on gluten withdrawal.

35　Stricturing can occur within weeks or months of ingestion. The lifetime risk of oesophageal malignancy is increased by 50 times.

36　(a) Chronic hepatitis B.
(b) Close contacts may require vaccination.

37　(a) Pancreatic calcification.
(b) Chronic pancreatitis.

38　(a) Melanosis coli.
(b) The patient may have been abusing laxatives.

39　Trophozoite of *Giardia lamblia*.

40   (a) There are multiple distended loops of small intestine containing air-fluid levels. Gas shadows within the biliary tree are visible in the right upper quadrant.
(b) This is gallstone ileus. A large gallstone has migrated from a fistula between inflamed gall bladder and small intestine, and has become impacted in the terminal ileum to cause small bowel obstruction.

41   Vitamin B12 deficiency giving rise to sore fissured tongue and peripheral neuropathy.

42   (a) Calcified pleural plaques.
(b) Industrial asbestos exposure can cause pleural calcification as well as mesothelioma of the pleura or peritoneum.

43   (a) Leiomyoma of the stomach.
(b) Sarcomatous change.
(c) Surgical wedge excision.

44   (a) Grey Turner's sign.
(b) Acute pancreatitis.
(c) Retroperitoneal haemorrhage.

45   (a) Multiple small gas filled submucosal spaces.
(b) Pneumatosis cystoides intestinalis (pneumatosis coli).
(c) Continuous high-flow oxygen.

46   (a) Leuconychia (white nails).
(b) Hypoalbuminaemia.
(c) Hepatic cirrhosis, nephrotic syndrome.

47, 48
(a) Behcet's syndrome.
(b) Genital ulceration, thrombophlebitis, uveitis, neurological manifestations.

49   (a) Carcinoma of the head of the pancreas.
(b) Endoscopic stent insertion or surgical biliary bypass.

50   (a) Hydatid cyst.
(b) Large cysts of this magnitude generally require surgical excision followed by treatment with albendazole.

51   Oesophageal dysmotility. The radiograph shows the typical 'corkscrew oesophagus'.

52   (a) Gastric antral vascular ectasia ('watermelon stomach').
(b) Conservative (lifelong iron supplementation), laser (time-consuming – has to be repeated frequently) or partial gastrectomy.

53, 54

(a) Thickened terminal ileum with narrowing and a cobblestone appearance to the mucosal surface.

(b) Crohn's disease.

(c) Transmural inflammation, fissure formation on the right, and pink-staining granulomas within lymphoid aggregates.

55, 56

(a) Calcinosis, ulceration of terminal digit from Raynaud's phenomenon, sclerodactyly.

(b) Oesophageal involvement, telangiectasia (CREST syndrome variant of systemic sclerosis).

57   (a) A large polyp of the sigmoid colon.

(b) Total colonoscopy to assess the lesion and to exclude synchronous polyps or carcinomas in the rest of the colon.

(c) The lesion may be amenable to colonoscopic snare polypectomy. A sigmoid colectomy should be recommended if the mucosa surrounding the polyp is involved, or if the histology of the polyp shows poorly differentiated carcinoma or the presence of malignancy at the excision margin.

58   (a) Ampullary tumour. A periampullary diverticulum is also present – an incidental finding.

(b) If biopsy confirms ampullary carcinoma the patient should be considered for Whipple's pancreaticoduodenectomy.

59   The sacro-iliac joints show periarticular sclerosis. The joint is almost fused on the left side. There is an association between sacro-ileitis and ulcerative colitis.

60   (a) Partial villous atrophy with crypt hyperplasia.

(b) Tropical sprue.

(c) Folic acid and tetracycline.

61   Mallory-Weiss tear. The picture was taken at the gastro-oesophageal junction. A congested fold with a mucosal tear is seen at 11 o'clock. This appearance is induced by copious vomiting.

62   Rotavirus gastroenteritis.

63   (a) There is dilatation of the left main hepatic duct, and filling defects are seen within the dilated area.

(b) Asiatic cholangiohepatitis due to clonorchiasis (Chinese liver flukes).

(c) Cholangiocarcinoma.

64   (a) Gross ascites, multiple spider naevi, dilated superficial veins.

(b) Hepatic cirrhosis.

65   (a) The mucosa is pale and the lesion has rolled edges. The most likely diagnosis is early gastric cancer.

(b) Partial gastrectomy is indicated if endoscopic biopsy confirms the diagnosis.

(c) Early gastric cancer, with invasion confined to the mucosa and submucosa, has a good prognosis.

66   (a) Radiolabelled leucocyte scan (white cells labelled with either ^{111}Indium or ^{99}Technetium HMPAO are re-injected intravenously and are taken up in inflamed bowel).

(b) Inflammatory bowel disease affecting most of the colon.

67, 68

(a) Hairy leucoplakia.

(b) Oocyst of *Isospora belli* in the centre of the field.

(c) AIDS.

69   (a) Massive splenic enlargement, osteosclerosis.

(b) Myelofibrosis

70   (a) Stigmata of recent bleeding (red spot in ulcer base) Duodenitis and scarring from previous silent ulceration.

(b) Testing for Helicobacter pylori. Alternatives are 13C-urea breath testing, or gastric antral mucosal biopsy for rapid urease test, histology or culture.

(c) Healing with acid–suppressing drugs with long-term maintenance therapy with histamine H_2 blockers is the traditional approach. Nowadays most patients receive eradication therapy against *H. pylori* to heal the ulcer and prevent recurrence.

71   Umbilical hernia complicated by strangulation.

72   (a) Percutaneous transhepatic cholangiogram.

(b) Cholangiocarcinoma affecting the bifurcation of the common hepatic duct (Klatskin tumour).

73   Orofacial granulomatosis (Melkersson-Rosenthal syndrome), Crohn's disease, sarcoidosis.

74   (a) Narrowing of sigmoid colon with cobblestone appearance and ulceration. A separate lesion (skip lesion) is seen in the distal transverse colon. There is pseudosacculation due to asymetrical patchy large bowel involvement and two large 'rosethorn' ulcers are seen.

(b) Crohn's disease.

75, 76
      (a) Primary gastric lymphoma.
      (b) Surgical – usually subtotal gastrectomy.

77   (a) ERCP.
      (b) Primary sclerosing cholangitis.
      (c) Ulcerative colitis.

78   (a) Exophthalmos, goitre.
      (b) Thyrotoxicosis.

79   (a) Replacement of the lower oesophageal epithelium by gastric columnar epithelium. The junction between the two types of mucosa is irregular.
      (b) Barrett's oesophagus.
      (c) Benign ulceration, stricture formation, malignant change.

80   Benign serous cystadenoma, cystadenocarcinoma.

81, 82
      (a) Villous adenoma.
      (b) Anterior resection or piecemeal colonoscopic polypectomy.

83   Colonic diverticular disease, colonic carcinoma, Crohn's disease, tuberculosis.

84   Neurofibromatosis (von Recklinghausen's disease). A Schwannoma is compressing the spinal cord or cauda equina interfering with the nerve supply to the anal sphincters.

85   (a) Carcinoma of the oesophagus (carcinoma of the bronchus less likely).
      (b) Tracheo-oesophageal fistula.
      (c) Endoscopic stent insertion.

86   Portal hypertensive gastropathy (congestive gastropathy).

87   (a) Perianal Crohn's disease (possible small abscess close to patient's left labia).
      (b) Metronidazole.

88   Large hiatus hernia with retrocardiac fluid level.

89   (a) Pseudomembranous colitis due to *Clostridium difficile* (antibiotic-associated colitis).
      (b) Oral vancomycin or metronidazole.
      (c) The patient should be barrier nursed in a cubicle because there is a cross-infection risk.

(b) Dehydration with hypochloraemic alkalosis.

91, 92

(a) Peutz-Jehgers syndrome.
(b) Small bowel intussusception.
(c) Gastrointestinal bleeding, increased cancer risk (gastrointestinal and extra-intestinal).

93 (a) Coeliac disease (gluten–sensitive enteropathy).
(b) Lymphoma of the small intestine, squamous carcinoma of the oropharynx or oesophagus.

94 (a) Angiodysplastic spot.
(b) Continued oral iron therapy. Endoscopic treatment is normally reserved for patients who develop recurrent anaemia despite iron.

95, 96

(a) Scattered ulceration from mid-sigmoid to transverse colon. Barium is seen to exit the narrowed mid-sigmoid colon into a track.
(b) Large abscess with air–fluid level.
(c) Percutaneous drainage under ultrasound guidance or surgical drainage, together with broad-spectrum antibiotics.

97 (a) Hereditary spherocytosis.
(b) Inherited as an autosomal dominant disorder.
(c) Biliary colic due to a pigment stone in the common bile duct.

98 (a) Smooth lateral margins of tongue with loss of papillae.
(b) Iron deficiency.

99 (a) Large oesophageal varices.
(b) White nipple sign (fibrin plaque), cherry red spots (red colour signs).

100 (a) Large left-sided hydropneumothorax with tension. The mediastinum is shifted to the right.
(b) Spontaneous rupture of the oesophagus (Boerhaave's syndrome).

101 Systemic sclerosis can affect the small intestine causing stasis and even pseudo-obstruction. Stasis predisposes to bacterial overgrowth and hence malabsorption.

102 (a) A roundworm (*Ascaris lumbricoides*) is present in the common bile duct.
(b) The worm may be removed and retrieved after endoscopic sphincterotomy; systemic antihelminthic drugs given.

103, 104

(a) Amoebic dysentery (one *Entamoeba histolytica* trophozoite containing ingested red cells is seen in the centre of the photomicrograph).

(b) Five to 10-day course of oral metronidazole, or single large oral dose of tinidazole.

105 (a) Multiple scratch marks.

(b) Phenothiazine-induced cholestasis.

(c) Discontinue offending drug, cholestyramine (an anion exchange resin) may relieve pruritus.

106 There is focal accumulation of tracer in the central abdomen. The gastric mucosa is also registering. These are the appearances of a Meckel's diverticulum.

107 (a) The ulcer may be the sign of a more serious disorder, such as carcinoma or lymphoma; the patient may not have been complying with drug treatment; or he may have an underlying gastrinoma causing the Zollinger-Ellison syndrome with gastric acid hypersecretion.

(b) Biopsy of the ulcer, fasting serum gastrin, basal acid output.

108 (a) Telangiectasia of the lips.

(b) Hereditary haemorrhagic telangiectasia.

(c) Recurrent epistaxis, anaemia, haemoptysis, upper or lower gastrointestinal bleeding.

109, 110

(a) Ileocaecal tuberculosis.

(b) Large caseating granuloma with occasional giant cells.

111 (a) Pyogenic liver abscess. Note the multiple cavities with surrounding ring enhancement after contrast.

(b) Broad-spectrum antibiotics and percutaneous drainage. Open surgical drainage should be considered if there is no clinical improvement.

112 Tylosis palmaris.

113, 114

(a) Haemobilia (blood clot is protruding from the ampulla and is demonstrated within the opacified biliary tree).

(b) An uncommon complication of liver biopsy.

115 (a) There is gross displacement of the greater curve of the stomach by an extrinsic mass.

(b) The mass is a pancreatic pseudocyst, confirmed by ultrasonography.

(c) The traditional treatment is surgical cystogastrostomy. The alternative technique is percutaneous endoscopic cystogastrostomy under radiological guidance.

116 (a) Fistula in ano.
(b) Although usually idiopathic, fistulae in ano may complicate Crohn's disease, tuberculosis or rectal carcinoma.

117 (a) Small bowel enema (enteroclysis).
(b) Several jejunal strictures with ulceration and areas of dilated bowel between strictures. The loops are widely separated suggesting bowel wall thickening.
(c) Small bowel Crohn's disease. Tuberculosis can give this appearance but more typically affects the ileum.

118 Glass eye enucleation of right eye for melanoma; after she has now developed multiple liver metastases.

119 (a) Gross dilatation of the ascending and transverse colon. This is likely to be due to toxic dilatation.
(b) Ulcerative colitis.
(c) Crohn's disease, infective colitis (especially Salmonella and pseudomembranous colitis). Chaga's disease can cause massive colonic dilatation, but large amounts of faecal residue are usually obvious.

120 (a) Secondary syphilis.
(b) Serological tests.

121 Pelvic abscess. The black/white air/fluid level is shown to the right side of the bowel lumen.

122 (a) Idiopathic haemochromatosis (note the 'slatey–grey' pigmentation).
(b) Weekly venesection until liver iron deposition has been cleared.
(c) Primary hepatocellular carcinoma.

123 Large oesophageal diverticulum containing food residue.

124 (a) Submucosal arterial malformation (Dieulafoy's lesion). The tip of a large blood vessel is protruding on the right side of the photograph. There is only minimal associated ulceration.
(b) Endoscopic treatment (e.g. alcohol injection) or surgical wedge resection. The chances of rebleeding are very high if no treatment is given.

125 (a) Sulphasalazine-induced pneumonitis.
(b) Sulphasalazine should be discontinued and a 5-amino salicylic acid drug used instead. Corticosteroids may be required.

126   (a) Psoriasis.
(b) Hepatic fibrosis due to methotrexate.

127   (a) There is gross retention of meconium proximal to the rectum.
(b) Hirschprung's disease.

128   (a) Complete rectal prolapse.
(b) Surgery – either internal pelvic fixation of rectum or perineal rectal excision.

129   (a) Gross irregular dilatation of the pancreatic duct with 'chain of lakes' appearance.
Pancreatic calcification is also obvious.
(b) Chronic pancreatitis.
(c) Alcohol.

130   (a) Pyoderma gangrenosum.
(b) Inflammatory bowel disease.
(c) Control of the underlying bowel disorder, usually with oral corticosteroids.
Occasionally resection of the affected bowel is indicated.

131, 132
(a) Linear calcification of menisci (chondrocalcinosis).
(b) Whipple's disease.

133   (a) Henoch-Schönlein purpura.
(b) Gastrointestinal bleeding, renal failure.

134   A neuroendocrine islet-cell tumour was producing gastrin which, in turn, stimulated massive gastric acid hypersecretion (Zollinger-Ellison syndrome).

135   (a) Previous surgery (choledochoduodenostomy, choledochojejunostomy).
(b) Ascending cholangitis.
(c) Reflux of small bowel contents into the biliary tree; a sump syndrome with stasis in the common bile duct distal to the anastomosis.

136   (a) Localised dilatation of the main pancreatic duct and its side branches in the tail of the pancreas.
(b) Chronic pancreatitis.

137, 138
(a) Granular haemorrhagic mucosa with mucus exudate.
(b) Ulcerative colitis.
(c) Biopsy helps to distinguish self-limited colitis (due to infectious agent, drug or unknown cause) from early inflammatory bowel disease. In this biopsy there is major disruption to the mucosal architecture with a villous morphology and dense

lymphocytic infiltrate. These features strongly suggest inflammatory bowel disease that is likely to pursue a chronic course.

139   (a) Episcleritis.
       (b) Inflammatory bowel disease.

140   (a) Looser's zones (pseudofractures of the pelvic rami).
       (b) Osteomalacia.
       (c) Malabsorption (e.g. coeliac disease), cholestatic liver disease, lack of sunlight or lack of dietary calcium or vitamin D.

141   Coeliac disease, Crohn's disease, ulcerative colitis, Whipple's disease, alpha chain disease, hepatic cirrhosis.

142   (a) Linitis plastica.
       (b) Gastric carcinoma.

143   (a) Elevation of right hemidiaphragm.
       (b) Subphrenic abscess. The anti-inflammatory drugs had suppressed the acute manifestations of intra-abdominal sepsis.

144   (a) Lichen planus.
       (b) Oesophageal ulceration and stricture formation.
       (c) A combination of corticosteroids and antisecretory drugs.

145, 146
       (a) Kaposi's sarcoma.
       (b) Numerous acid–alcohol fast bacilli.
       (c) AIDS.

147, 148
       (a) Squamous carcinoma of the oesophagus.
       (b) External or endoluminal radiotherapy (brachytherapy); endoscopic intubation, laser or alcohol injection.

149   (a) Loss of haustration and ulceration of colon with multiple pseudopolyps. There is sparing of the rectum and ascending colon.
       (b) Corticosteroid enema therapy.

150   (a) Carcinoid syndrome.
       (b) Estimation of 24-h urinary 5-hydroxyindolacetic acid excretion together with demonstration of carcinoid tumour (e.g. ultrasound-guided liver biopsy).

151   (a) Enterocolic fistula.
       (b) Carcinoma of the colon.

(c) Bacterial overgrowth of the small intestine.

152 (a) Inflammatory bowel disease, especially Crohn's disease.
(b) Sigmoidoscopy (or colonoscopy) and biopsy, barium studies, technetium-labelled leucocyte scanning (see **66**).

153 (a) Urease test.
(b) The sample turning red is urease positive. This patient has gastritis due to *Helicobacter pylori*. The other patient is probably negative, although drugs, including antibiotics, can cause a falsely negative result.
(c) Duodenal or gastric ulcers found during endoscopy.

154 (a) Narrowing and mucosal oedema (thumb printing) of the splenic flexure and proximal descending colon.
(b) Ischaemic colitis.
(c) Benign stricture formation.

155 (a) Anal carcinoma.
(b) Abdominoperineal resection.

156 (a) Dilatation of the biliary tree with narrowing and lateral displacement of lower end of common bile duct. Calcification in the head of the pancreas is also seen.
(b) Chronic pancreatitis.

157, 158
(a) Free perforation of the jejunum.
(b) Drug-induced; non-steroidal anti-inflammatory drugs are likely to be implicated in this case.

159 (a) Eruptive xanthomas.
(b) Familial hypertriglyceridaemia.
(c) Recurrent acute pancreatitis.

160 Small bowel obstruction from strangulated hernia. An extraperitoneal gas shadow from the entrapped small bowel within the hernia sac is seen at the bottom of the film.

161, 162
(a) Transition from inflamed mucosa at the left of the field to severe dysplasia at the right.
(b) Malignant change.
(c) Total colectomy, with permanent ileostomy or ileoanal pouch construction.

163 Pyostomatitis vegetans.

164 (a) Selective superior mesenteric angiography.
(b) Angiodysplasia of caecum and, perhaps, terminal ileum.

165, 166
(a) Schistosomiasis.
(b) Liver involvement with portal hypertension.

167 (a) Gastric erosions.
(b) Aspirin therapy.

168 (a) Pharyngeal pouch (Zenker's diverticulum).
(b) Aspiration pneumonia.
(c) No. Endoscopy has little or nothing to add and is potentially hazardous –
inadvertent intubation of the diverticulum could lead to perforation.
(d) Surgical excision of the pouch.

169, 170
(a) Thrombosis and disruption of an arteriole at the bottom of the field.
(b) Vasculitis.
(c) Anti-neutrophil cytoplasmic antibody (ANCA) test.

171 (a) Macronodular cirrhosis, hepatocellular carcinoma.
(b) Chronic viral hepatitis (B or C).

172
(a) Percutaneous transhepatic cholangiography.
(b) Cholangiocarcinoma, carcinoma of the gall bladder, or extrinsic compression
by tumour or enlarged lymph nodes. This patient turned out to have an impacted
gallstone at the junction of cystic and common hepatic ducts (Mirizzi syndrome).

173, 174
(a) Erythema nodosum.
(b) Mucosal erythema, loss of vascular pattern, cobblestone mucosa.
(c) Crohn's colitis.

175, 176
(a) A very large spider naevus.
(b) Fatty change, infiltration with polymorphonuclear leucocytes, occasional liver
cell necrosis with red-staining alcoholic hyaline.
(c) Alcoholic liver disease.

177 (a) There is gas in the soft tissues of the neck. There is a small amount of
subpulmonary gas and a small right pleural effusion. A central venous catheter is
present.

(b) She has oesophageal perforation from endoscopy. She should remain nil by mouth for several days. Analgesia, antibiotics and nutritional support should be given parenterally. Surgery may be required in the event of continuing deterioration.

178 (a) Peristomal varices.
(b) Portal hypertension from sclerosing cholangitis.

179 (a) Ischiorectal abscess.
(b) Antibiotics and early operative drainage.

180 Barrett's oesophagus complicated by malignant change.

181 (a) There is a blue line at the margin of gums and teeth.
(b) Lead poisoning.

182 (a) Dilatation of the oesophagus, some hold-up of barium above a narrowed lower oesophagus, indentations and tapering of the lower oesophagus. These are the characteristic features of achalasia.
(b) Oesophageal manometry. Endoscopy to exclude malignancy.

183 (a) Pseudoxanthoma elasticum.
(b) The retina, which may show angioid streaks.
(c) Vascular degeneration in the gut.

184 Neurological dysphagia secondary to stroke or bulbar palsy (motor–neurone disease, amyotrophic lateral sclerosis). Malignancy (head, neck, pharyngeal or oesophageal cancer).

185 (a) Intravariceal injection sclerotherapy.
(b) Local necrosis with ulceration; stricture formation; introduction of infection (several sequelae described).
(c) Rubber band ligation.

186 (a) Oedematous and empty colon with loss of haustral folds. The folds in the transverse colon are grossly thickened.
(b) Colitis – probably extensive ulcerative colitis.

187 (a) Degos' disease (malignant atrophic papulosis).
(b) Intestinal perforation.

188 (a) Left-sided supraclavicular lymphadenopathy.
(b) Carcinoma of the oesophagus or stomach.

189 (a) Areas of hypertrophy of retinal pigment epithelium.

(b) Familial adenomatous polyposis, especially Gardner's syndrome.

190 (a) Mucosal irregularity and ulceration extending from the caecum to the splenic flexure. Note that the appendix is also involved.
(b) Crohn's disease.

191 (a) Greenish–brown ring of copper-containing pigment at the periphery of the cornea.
(b) Wilson's disease (hepaticolenticular degeneration).
(c) Patients may present with symptoms of chronic active hepatitis, such as jaundice. Alternatively, neurological features (e.g. movement disorders, dysarthria or behavioural disturbances) may predominate. Haemolytic anaemia is a third possible presenting feature.

192 Hepatitis B, and possibly superimposed delta (hepatitis D). Hepatitis C virus infection is even more likely. There is now evidence that intravenous drug users can become infected with hepatitis G.

193 (a) Pericardial calcification.
(b) Constrictive pericarditis (probably from tuberculosis).

Index